Color
Atlas of
Pediatric
Dermatology

Color Atlas of
Pediatric Dermatology

Second Edition

Samuel Weinberg, M.D., F.A.A.P., F.A.C.P.

Clinical Professor of Dermatology
New York University Medical Center
New York, New York

Neil S. Prose, M.D., F.A.A.P.

Assistant Professor of Dermatology and Pediatrics
State University of New York
Health Science Center at Brooklyn
Brooklyn, New York

Histopathology by Lewis Shapiro, M.D.

Formerly Professor of Clinical Dermatology
  and Clinical Pathology
College of Physicians and Surgeons
Columbia University
New York, New York

McGraw-Hill Information Services Company

HEALTH PROFESSIONS DIVISION

New York St. Louis San Francisco Colorado Springs Auckland Bogotá Caracas Hamburg
Lisbon London Madrid Mexico Milan Montreal New Delhi Paris San Juan São Paulo
Singapore Sydney Tokyo Toronto

Color Atlas of Pediatric Dermatology

1234567890   KGPKGP   89432109

ISBN   0-07-069089-8

This book was set in Times Roman by Monotype Composition Co., Inc.
The editors were Avé M. McCracken and Muza Navrozov;
the production supervisor was Clare B. Stanley;
the cover was designed by Jose Fonfrias;
the index was prepared by Robert Zolnerzack.
Color work was done by Lehigh Colortronics.
Arcata Graphics/Kingsport was printer and binder.

Library of Congress Cataloging-in-Publication Data

Weinberg, Samuel, date.
    Color atlas of pediatric dermatology / Samuel Weinberg, Neil S.
Prose; histopathology by Lewis Shapiro. — 2nd ed.
      p. cm.
    Includes index.
    ISBN 0-07-069089-8
    1. Pediatric dermatology—Atlases. I. Prose, Neil S.
II. Shapiro, Lewis. III. Title.
    [DNLM: 1. Skin Diseases—in infancy & childhood—atlases. WS 17
W423c]
RJ511.W44 1990
618.92′5′0222—dc20
DNLM/DLC
for Library of Congress   89-12373
                              CIP

Credits for Photographs

Arturo Aballi
A. Bernard Ackerman
J. O'D. Alexander
William G. Ballinger
Charles S. Baraf
Alexander G. Bearn
Jerrold M. Becker
Bernard W. Berger
Eugene L. Bodian
Martin H. Brownstein
Philip Charney
Platon J. Collipp
Maurice J. Costello
Vincent Derbes
Anthony N. Domonkos
Leon Eisenbud
Robert P. Feinstein
Ilona J. Frieden
Alexander A. Fisher

Robert W. Goltz
Ralph W. Grover
Paul Honig
Jonathan Horwitz
Sidney Hurwitz
Kathleen L. Hussey
Josef E. Jelinek
S. Wayne Klein
Irwin H. Krasna
Jose Kriner
Saul Krugman
Teresita A. Laude
Chester M. Lessenden, Jr.
Luther B. Lowe
John McSorley
Lamar S. Osment
John R. T. Reeves
Perry Robins
Victor Torres Rodriguez

Avron Ross
James P. Rotchford
Wiley M. Sams
Arthur Sawitsky
Lawrence A. Schachner
Keith M. Schneider
Edward Shapiro
Meyer H. Slatkin
Roy Stephens
Conrad Stritzler
Ronald Stritzler
Joel A. Teisch
Louis Tobin
Donald Waldorf
William A. Welton
Zelma Wessely
Constance Y. Wong
Alex W. Young, Jr.
Erwin Zimmerman

Department of Dermatology, College of Physicians and Surgeons, Columbia University

New York University School of Medicine (Skin and Cancer Unit) permitted use of photographs for the following figures: 14, 53, 62, 66, 84, 161, 163, 198, 207, 208, 209, 212, 214, 217, 221, 257, 294, 295, 296, 302, 304, 308, 309, 324, 328, 329, 336, 339, 345, 357, 362, 363, 370, 372, 393, 408, 421, 423, 426, 429, 437, 440, 481, 514, 555, 574, 592, 639, 659, 682, 709, 737, 748, 762, 764, 769, 779, 781

The following figures have been used with permission:

Figure 247: I. J. Frieden, N. S. Prose, V. Fletcher, and M. L. Turner, "Granulomatous Perioral Dermatitis in Children." Copyright © 1989, American Medical Association. *Archives of Dermatology* 125:369–373, 1989. **Figures 430** and **431:** Ilona J. Frieden and Nancy B. Esterly, "Selected Granulomatoses in Infants and Children." Copyright © 1988 by Lippincott/Harper & Row. *Clinics in Dermatology,* Vol. 3, No. 1, Jan.–Mar., 1988, p. 22. **Figures 534, 539,** and **540:** *Journal of the American Academy of Dermatology* (in press). **Figure 535:** *Pediatric Dermatology* 4:67–74, 1987. **Figures 536** and **538:** *Advances in Dermatology* (in press).

Contents

Section 14   Bullous, Pustular, and Ulcerating Diseases   Page 139

Section 15   Cutaneous Manifestations of Systemic Disease   Page 149

Preface

The twelve years since the first edition of this color atlas have witnessed an explosion of knowledge in the field of pediatric dermatology. Pediatric dermatology has matured into a respected discipline, with its own diagnostic approaches and modes of therapy. This change has been highlighted by the creation of British, American, and international societies for pediatric dermatology and of journals and textbooks devoted exclusively to this field.

The primary purposes in undertaking this new edition have been to update the descriptions of previously recognized cutaneous diseases and to include more than 20 dermatoses that were not previously described. Most of these were unknown when the first edition was written.

Examples of these newly included entities are such major illnesses as Lyme disease, Kawasaki's disease, and neonatal lupus erythematosus. Examples of other "new" and important cutaneous conditions are transient neonatal pustular melanosis, chronic bullous disease of childhood, and congenital candidiasis.

In addition, a section on the cutaneous manifestations of human immunodeficiency virus (HIV) infection in children has been added. The mucocutaneous diseases that are seen more frequently among children with AIDS and lesser forms of HIV infection are illustrated here. Thanks go to the Society for Pediatric Dermatology for funding the research which made some of these photographs possible.

The text of the second edition of the atlas bears the indelible imprint of Dr. Morris Leider, a co-author of the first edition. Dr. Leider died in 1986 after a long illness. His warmth, wit, dermatologic knowledge, and dedication to the precise and imaginative use of the English language can be appreciated in the several passages that have been left intact. The connoisseur of his unique writing style will immediately recognize his continued literary influence in the humorous discussions of insect "bites" and branchial-cleft cysts.

The format of this atlas allows for only a brief discussion of the etiology and clinical appearance of each disease entity. We have also tried to include some very basic therapeutic suggestions. We ask the reader to bear in mind that this volume is not a textbook and that it should be used in conjunction with one of the several comprehensive references on pediatric dermatology. It is our hope that this atlas will be of practical use to all health practitioners who are involved in the care of children.

Color
Atlas of
Pediatric
Dermatology

1

Benign Neonatal Dermatoses

Figure 1

Figure 2

Erythema toxicum neonatorum This very common and completely benign condition usually arises in the first 2 days of life. It is seen in about half of healthy newborns and occurs less frequently in preterm infants. The lesions are erythematous macules, within which papules and pustules may develop. The trunk is the most common site, but all other body surfaces, except for the palms and soles, may be involved. The eruption in Fig. 1 began 2 hours after delivery and involved the face and trunk. The eruption in Fig. 2 was

unusual in that it was so widespread and vesiculopustular. Occasionally, this unimportant eruption must be differentiated from more serious infectious processes, such as neonatal herpes simplex. Tzanck smear of a pustule of erythema toxicum neonatorum will reveal numerous eosinophils but no multinucleated giant cells or bacteria. Occasionally, peripheral eosinophilia is also present. The cause of this condition is not known, and it resolves spontaneously within 10 days. No treatment is required.

Figure 3

Figure 4

Transient neonatal pustular melanosis This is a benign neonatal dermatosis that is most common among black infants. The original lesion is a vesiculopustule, which may be present at birth. This small blister quickly ruptures and leaves a typical collarette of superficial scale. Both intact pustules and collarettes are seen in the newborn in Fig. 3. Figure 4 shows the brownish pigmented macules that develop at the site of each resolving pustule. These macules may be sparse or numerous and resolve without residua over a period of several weeks to several months. In some infants, the pustule

and collarette stages seem to occur in utero, and the sole cutaneous manifestations are the typical macules. Lesions of transient neonatal pustular melanosis favor the forehead, neck, chin, and lower back but may be very widespread and may involve the palms and soles. Scraping the base of an unroofed pustule reveals polymorphonuclear leukocytes but no bacteria, pseudohyphae, or multinucleated giant cells. A biopsy of a pustule, which is rarely necessary, shows an intraepidermal collection of polymorphonuclear leukocytes.

2

Milia, Miliaria, and Pustular and Acneiform Disorders

Figure 5

Figure 6

Milia A milium is a white papule, 1–2 mm in size, composed of laminated, keratinous material and situated as a solid cyst in a pilosebaceous follicle. Milia are fairly common on the brow, glabella, and nose in newborn infants and in such infants tend to disappear quickly and spontaneously. There may be few or many, and they may develop later in infancy, in childhood, and in adolescence. In older children and adolescents, they tend to persist, may foretell acne or be associated with incipient acne, and commonly develop on or about the eyelids. Milia may be ablated, if desirable, by delicate incision and expression of their keratinous content. Lesions so treated do not recur, but if new lesions appear, they have to be treated in the same way. The operation is trivial and uncomplicated. There are no preventive measures. When acne is associated, it is the more serious and difficult condition to manage.

Figure 7

Figure 8

Eosinophilic pustular folliculitis of infancy Children with this rare disorder develop repeated crops of pruritic yellow or white pustules which vary in size from 1 to 3 mm. Most lesions are located on the scalp and distal extremities. Tzanck smear reveals numerous eosinophils, and there may also be a peripheral eosinophilia. Eosinophilic pustular folliculitis is associated with no systemic symptoms and eventually resolves spontaneously. Therapy with mild topical steroids is somewhat beneficial.

Infantile acropustulosis This cutaneous disorder is characterized by recurrent episodes of intensely pruritic pustules and papulovesicles on the hands and feet. Lesions are most common on the palms and soles but may be seen on the dorsal surfaces as well. The age of onset is typically between the ages of 2 and 10 months, and the disease resolves spontaneously by 2 to 3 years of age. The episodes of recurrence may occur as often as every 2 weeks at the beginning of the disease and tend to become less frequent and severe over time.

Figure 9

Figure 10

Miliaria crystallina The lesions in this condition are small, clear, thin-roofed vesicles that develop when the sweat duct is obstructed within the stratum corneum. They occur after sunburn or in response to excessive sweating in high environmental heat and humidity. Fever may also be a cause. The scalp, face, trunk, and intertriginous areas are sites of lesions. Itching is not a symptom. The vesicles resolve rapidly with the elimination of the causative environmental factor.

Miliaria rubra (prickly heat) This is the most common form of miliaria. It occurs when there is plugging of the eccrine ducts within the malpighian layer and release of sweat into the adjacent skin. Miliaria rubra is characterized by discrete erythematous papules and papulovesicles. The forehead, upper trunk, and intertriginous areas are commonly affected. Unlike miliaria crystallina, miliaria rubra is characterized by spasmodic pricking sensations. A decrease in environmental heat and humidity is the only treatment required.

Figure 11

Figure 12

Miliaria pustulosa Progression from miliaria rubra to miliaria pustulosa is related to duration of sweat duct occlusion, the amount of sweat retention, and the degree of inflammation around the ducts. In affected patients, one sees the typical erythematous papules of miliaria rubra, and, in addition, lesions which are frankly pustular. Although this condition may resemble a bacterial pyoderma, it responds well to the appropriate adjustment in environmental heat and humidity.

Multiple sweat-gland abscesses (miliaria profunda) The forms of miliaria described above are limited to the portion of the sweat apparatus within the epidermis. Occasionally, obstruction of deeper portions of the sweat glands (the dermal ducts and coils) results in spillage of sweat into the dermis, inflammation, and secondary infection. The resultant abscesses are firm and are slow to resolve by spontaneous rupture and discharge to the surface.

Figure 13

Figure 14

Fox-Fordyce disease (apocrine miliaria) This chronic and intensely pruritic papular eruption is localized to the axillae, areolae, and pubic areas. It occurs almost exclusively in young women, frequently with onset during adolescence. The follicular papules result from the obstruction of the intra-epidermal sweat duct, with release of apocrine sweat into the surrounding skin. Figure 13 shows the process in an axilla; Fig. 14 shows it in the pubic area. The etiology of Fox-Fordyce disease is unknown, and treatment is difficult. Topical and intralesional corticosteroids, estrogen therapy, and antimicrobial therapy are sometimes helpful.

Figure 15

Histopathology of Fox-Fordyce disease In miliaria of eccrine sweat glands, the histologic feature is a vesicle or pustule in the epidermis along the course of the sweat duct. In Fox-Fordyce disease (apocrine miliaria), such a lesion is found at a high level of a hair follicle because apocrine sweat ducts enter hair follicles rather than course directly to the surface as eccrine ducts do. Two vesicles so placed and containing inflammatory cells are seen in the photomicrograph. The underlying cutis is somewhat inflamed.

Figure 16

Figure 17

Neonatal and infantile acne   Mild comedonal acne is fairly common in the newborn. The typical eruption consists of closed comedones. Open comedones, inflammatory papules and pustules, and small cysts may also occur. Neonatal acne is attributed to the stimulation of sebaceous glands by androgens from both mother and infant. The lesions of neonatal acne usually resolve during the first few months of life. Acne, in varying degrees of severity, may also appear in infants after the newborn period. This form of infantile acne may persist for one or two years and may rarely eventuate in scarring. Children with early onset of acne and a strong family history are particulary at risk for a severe course of the disease during puberty. Most cases of neonatal and infantile acne do not require treatment. If necessary, a mild benzoyl peroxide may be used.

Figure 18

Figure 19

Acne vulgaris   The common varieties of acne generally begin to develop in late childhood or early adolescence. The earliest lesions are open or closed comedones, and these may progress to inflammatory papules, pustules, and cysts. Figure 18 shows the comedo stage; Fig. 19, the beginning of progression to inflammatory papules and pustules. Acne during adolescence is caused by the effect of androgenic hormones on the pilosebaceous unit. The increased activity of the sebaceous gland provides a substrate for *Proprynebacterium acnes*, whose lipolytic enzymes convert triglycerides in sebum to free fatty acids. This primary irritant causes the formation of comedones. Abnormal keratinization in the pilosebaceous follicle also plays a role in the development of acne. Topical therapies are aimed at decreasing skin colonization by *P. acnes* (topical antibiotics) and at normalizing keratinization within the follicle (tretinoin).

Figure 20

Cystic acne   Many cases of acne progress from open and closed comedones (blackheads and whiteheads) to inflammatory forms that are marked by papules, pustules, and cysts. Figure 20 shows a combination of these. Severe cystic acne is more difficult to control or cure and causes scarring. Topical therapy with combinations of antibiotics and tretinoin is of value. In addition, systemic antibiotics, such as tetracycline and erythromycin, are useful because of their antibacterial and anti-inflammatory properties. The intralesional injection of corticosteroids may also be helpful.

Figure 21

Acne conglobata   In conglobate acne, the most severe form of acne, cysts tend to be large, irregular, and intercommunicating, and to result in severe scarring. Severe cystic acne can sometimes be controlled with topical therapy and systemic antibiotics. The patient who does not respond to these measures may be a candidate for 13-*cis*-retinoic acid. Side effects of this therapy range from dry lips and skin to elevation of cholesterol and triglycerides. In addition, all female patients must be advised that 13-*cis*-retinoic acid is a potent teratogen and that pregnancy must be avoided.

Figure 22

Keloids following acne   Hypertrophic scars and keloids following resolution of inflammatory lesions of acne are an uncommon but particularly distressing complication. The chest and upper back are sites of predilection. Keloids occur less commonly on the face. The tendency toward keloid formation is more common in black adolescents and is sometimes familial. Successful control of the acne itself, through topical or systemic therapy, will minimize the extent of future scarring. The use of intralesional corticosteroids is the most effective treatment of keloids once they have formed.

Figure 23

Acne and precocious puberty from a pinealoma   In this four-year-old child, persistent acne, precocious puberty, and frequent headache were the presenting signs and symptoms of a pinealoma. Occasionally, acne in a preadolescent may be an indication of an endocrine abnormality in which either androgen or glucocorticoids are present in excess. For example, a typical eruption of monomorphic follicular papules, usually concentrated on the back and chest, is seen in Cushing's disease. The same type of acne occurs in children undergoing systemic steroid therapy for any reason.

Figure 24

Figure 25

Hidradenitis suppurativa This condition is a chronic, recurrent inflammatory process of unknown etiology which involves the apocrine sweat glands. The favored locations are the axillae, groin, and buttocks. The disease begins just before or during puberty, and persists, with remissions and exacerbations, for years. It is more common in women and is sometimes associated with acne conglobata and dissecting cellulitis of the scalp. Worsening of the disease may be seen during summer months or at the time of menstruation.

Hidradenitis suppurativa is aggravated by obesity. Apocrine gland occlusion in the involved axilla or groin leads to the formation of pustules, nodules, abscesses, and sinus tracts. The disease process is complicated by chronic overgrowth with *Staphylococcus aureus* and a wide variety of anaerobes and gram-negative bacteria. The process pictured in Fig. 24 is situated in the anogenital region and is not particularly severe. The patient in Fig. 25 has more severe disease in the axilla.

Figure 26

Figure 27

Hidradenitis suppurativa In this photograph, the condition has partially, and temporarily, abated. Corded hypertrophic and keloidal scarring has developed. The treatment of hidradenitis suppurativa is often difficult. Topical and systemic antibiotics are most commonly used; the choice of an agent should be guided by repeated culture and sensitivities of the organisms in the purulent exudate. Intralesional steroids, incision and drainage of abscesses, and even surgical excision of the involved area are sometimes indicated.

Histopathology of hidradenitis suppurativa This condition starts as an acute suppurative, inflammatory process involving the secretory coils of the apocrine sweat glands. These are normally situated deep in the dermis and subcutaneous fat of the axillae, mammary areolae, and groin. In this photomicrograph one can see collections of inflammatory cells within the lumen of an apocrine sweat gland, surrounding it and traversing the epithelium of its coil (upper left and lower right corners).

Figure 28

Figure 29

Folliculitis et perifolliculitis capitis abscedens et suffodiens   This imposing title translates as an inflammation in and around hair follicles of the scalp that flows (pus) and channels under or through (tissue). A less imposing title is dissecting cellulitis of the scalp. This chronic condition resembles, and sometimes accompanies, acne conglobata and hidradenitis suppurativa (the follicular occlusion triad). Like them, it is marked by inflammation, purulence, intercommunicating abscesses, cysts

and sinuses, and scarring. This disease appears to be somewhat more common among blacks, and onset may occur during adolescence. A number of therapies are routinely used. These include topical and systemic antibiotics, incision and drainage of abscesses, and intralesional steroids. There are usually many remissions and exacerbations, and the process often eventuates in a scarring alopecia.

Figure 30

Figure 31

Acne varioliformis (acne necrotica)   This condition is characterized by recurrent, small, follicular papules, and pustules. The most common locations are the forehead and scalp. The lesions arise in crops and are initially painful or intensely pruritic. They umbilicate, ulcerate and crust, and the final result is numerous varioliform scars. Histologically, one sees intrafollicular subcorneal pustules and a perifollicular infiltrate.

Histopathology of folliculitis et perifolliculitis capitis abscedens et suffodiens   This condition (also known as dissecting cellulitis of the scalp) and acne keloidalis show an identical picture of inflammation and subsequent destruction of hair follicles. Dense scar tissue lacking elastic fibers subsequently forms. In the photomicrograph, one sees a partially destroyed follicle, inflammation, and scar tissue, with residual elastica only at the lower left.

Bacterial Infections

Figure 32

Figure 33

Impetigo contagiosa (vulgaris)   Impetigo is a primary super-ficial infection of the skin. It is more prevalent in humid climates and occurs most commonly in the summer months. Trauma to the skin, such as a small abrasion or insect bite, sometimes provides the site of entry for the infective bacteria. The lesions evolve from discrete small vesicles into pustules. The fluid content of the primary lesions dries into a thick, yellowish crust (Fig. 32), and removal of the crust may reveal bright, red, and shiny erosions (Fig. 33). The causative

streptococcus has been associated with epidemics of impetigo-induced acute glomerulonephritis. Because the "honey-crusted" lesions of impetigo are frequently caused by a combination of *Staphylococcus aureus* and *Streptococcus pyogenes,* systemic antibiotic therapy should be effective against both organisms. Topical mupirocin ointment appears to be an effective treatment and may replace the need for systemic therapy in some patients with localized lesions.

Figure 34

Figure 35

Bullous impetigo   This form of impetigo consists of flaccid blisters which quickly rupture and evolve into superficial, round or oval erosions with a varnished surface and minimal crust. Blisters are caused by the local effect of staphylococcal toxin. Pictured here are lesions in varying stages of evolution. Bullous impetigo is associated with a pure culture of *Staphylococcus aureus*. Oral treatment with dicloxacillin, eryth-romycin, or a cephalosporin is an effective mode of therapy.

Histopathology of impetigo contagiosa   In the common form of impetigo, whether caused by a pathogenic staphylococcus or streptococcus or both together, a subcorneal vesicle or bulla is produced as the initial or primary lesion. Neutrophils migrate through the living cellular portion of the epidermis (the stratum malpighii) and accumulate between it and the overlying, dead cornified portion (the stratum corneum). In the photomicrograph one sees intact and degenerating leu-kocytes together with epithelial debris in a pustule.

Figure 36

Figure 37

Staphylococcal scalded skin syndrome This eruption occurs most commonly in children under the age of 5. It is characterized by a generalized tender, macular erythema which is most prominent on the skin around the mouth and nose, and in intertriginous areas. Within 1 or 2 days, the rash begins to peel. Typically, the large superficial flaccid bullae ("scalded skin") are quickly unroofed, revealing areas of slightly erythematous and shiny skin. These areas crust and then heal. Children with this syndrome are often extremely irritable and febrile, but the overall prognosis is good. Figure 36 shows the typical crusting and fissuring around the lips and nose, and Fig. 37 illustrates superficial blistering on the buttock. The scalded skin syndrome is caused by an epidermolytic toxin which may be produced by several strains of *Staphylococcus aureus*. These causative organisms may be present in the nose, throat, conjunctiva, or an infected wound. Staphylococcal scalded skin syndrome resolves without scarring within a period of two weeks. Treatment consists of appropriate supportive care and penicillinase-resistant antibiotics.

Figure 38

Figure 39

Staphylococcal scalded skin syndrome The staphylococcal toxin exfoliatin may sometimes produce extensive areas of desquamation. Infants with this degree of involvement must be managed carefully with respect to fluid and electrolytes and must also receive topical therapy to minimize the risk of cutaneous infection by other organisms. Scalded skin syndrome must be differentiated from scarlet fever, Kawasaki's disease, toxic shock syndrome, and drug-induced toxic epidermal necrolysis.

Ecthyma Impetigo vulgaris is the most superficial of pyodermas; ecthyma is the next grade in depth. If impetigo is infection by streptococci and/or staphylococci superficially in the epidermis, ecthyma is infection by the same organisms through the entire thickness of the epidermis (0.1 mm) to the upper reaches of the dermis or "true skin" (perhaps to a depth of 0.5 mm). The lesion of ecthyma then becomes not a bulla but a firm crust on a superficial ulcer, surrounded by erythema.

Figure 40

Figure 41

Impetiginization This is the term for superficial pyoderma imposed upon preexisting dermatosis. Eruptions that are pruritic are particularly susceptible to secondary infection. Scratching disrupts the integrity of the epidermal barrier to infection and implants bacteria into the area of denuded skin. The most common organisms are *Streptococcus pyogenes* and *Staphylococcus aureus*. Pictured here is a case of impetiginized atopic dermatitis. The development of such "honey-crusted" lesions in a child with eczema suggests the need for antibiotic therapy.

Pyoderma complicating a thermal burn Secondary infection is a feared complication of thermal burns. Depending upon the extent and depth of a burn and on the infecting microorganism, pyodermatous complication may vary from trivial to life-threatening. *Pseudomonas aeruginosa* and mixed infections are the most difficult to overcome. In the patient pictured the burn was limited to the face, and the infecting organism was susceptible to antibiotics. The consequence was scarring, mostly from the burn.

Figure 42

Figure 43

Infectious eczematoid dermatitis This title should be reserved for that superficial inflammatory condition of the skin caused by pus overrunning from a nearby source. It is common from the nostril down on the upper lip from chronic nasal discharge, on the pinna of the ear from the meatus outward where there has been a run of pus from otitis externa, and around draining sinuses from a process like mastoiditis or osteomyelitis.

Chancriform pyoderma It sometimes happens that infection with a banal organism like a staphylococcus, or more often with organisms like *Pseudomonas aeruginosa* or a species of the genus *Proteus* and combinations thereof, results in chancriform ulcers. Such conditions are more difficult to cure than the usual run of pyodermatous ulcers. In addition to effective systemic antibiotics, wet dressings, adequate drainage, and topical antiseptics may be required.

Figure 44

Figure 45

Furuncle   A *furuncle* is a skin abscess or boil. Lesions of this type are usually caused by a coagulase-positive *Staphylococcus aureus*. The organism invades through either an area of damaged skin, a hair follicle, or a sebaceous gland. As bacteria multiply, a deep cavity containing polymorphonuclear leukocytes and bacteria is formed. Here pictured, in Fig. 44, is a furuncle on the chest and, in Fig. 45, on the labia. Abscesses can form anywhere on the body but are most common on the extremities, neck, buttocks, and axillae.

A *carbuncle* is a multiloculated abscess that forms when two or more neighboring furuncles become confluent. Many individuals with recurrent furuncles are found to be harboring the causative strain of *S. aureus* in the nares. Rarely, recurrent furunculosis is a sign of an underlying immune deficiency. In the earliest stages, intermittent warm compresses and systemic antibiotics may abort or mature lesions quickly. When lesions have pointed, incision and drainage is the treatment of choice.

Figure 46

Figure 47

Facial cellulitis   Cellulitis of the face may present in young children with a pink-to-purple edematous and warm discoloration of the cheek. In these cases, etiology is often *Hemophilus influenzae* or *Streptococcus pneumoniae*. There is usually high fever and toxicity, and often a preceding history of an otitis media. Complications of this form of infection include meningitis and sepsis. Rapid antibiotic therapy is mandatory, and the choice of antibiotic can be revised on the basis of blood and tissue aspirate cultures.

Erysipelas   This is a rare form of superficial cellulitis caused by group A β-hemolytic streptococci. Erysipelas frequently occurs on the face, and presents as a tense, warm, tender erythematous plaque with a well-demarcated border. The patient may be severely ill, with fever and local lymphadenopathy. Parenteral penicillin is often required in the initial, acute phase.

Figure 48

Figure 49

Scarlet fever Scarlet fever is a generalized exanthem of childhood, with the highest incidence between the ages of 2 and 10. The cause is infection of the oropharynx by group A β-hemolytic streptococcus. The rash results from an erythrogenic toxin produced by this bacteria. The disease begins after a short incubation period of 2–4 days with a pharyngitis, fever, and malaise. The skin then begins to show a diffuse punctate erythema, which has a fine "sandpaper" texture. The face may become flushed but not as erythematous as does the body (Fig. 48). Characteristically, there is pallor

around the mouth and tip of the nose. Erythema is deepest in skin folds, especially the antecubital fossae and axillary lines. Petechiae in linear arrangement (Pastia's lines) may develop. Tender, cervical adenopathy is usual. A red pharynx, purulent tonsillitis, strawberry tongue, and palatal petechiae may also be present. Desquamation of the hands, feet, elbows, and knees occurs during healing. Occasionally, peeling in these locations may be the sole cutaneous manifestation of a mild, resolving streptococcal infection.

Figure 50

Figure 51

Perianal streptococcal disease Group A β-hemolytic streptococcus is sometimes the cause of perianal inflammation in a child. This localized infection is accompanied by painful defecation or pruritus. Examination of the area reveals a bright-red erythema surrounding the rectum and oozing from the infected area of skin. Diagnosis may be confirmed by perianal swab and culture, and treatment consists of oral penicillin.

Blistering distal dactylitis This is a distinctive cutaneous infection that is caused by group A β-hemolytic streptococcus. The clinical appearance, as illustrated here, is a superficial blister over the anterior fat pad of the distal phalanx. One or more fingers may be involved. The blister fluid is culture-positive for the causative bacteria, and treatment consists of incision and drainage, along with the appropriate antibiotic by mouth.

Figure 52

Figure 53

Cat-scratch disease This disease is characterized by the appearance of a papule or pustule at the site of a scratch from a cat. Within several weeks, enlarged regional lymph nodes (Fig. 52) develop and become tender and fluctuant. Cat-scratch disease is accompanied by fever and malaise in about one-third of cases. Localized adenopathy may last from several weeks to months and then resolves spontaneously. Central nervous system involvement is a very rare but sometimes serious complication. A gram-negative bacterium has been isolated from involved lymph nodes.

Actinomycosis This is a chronic granulomatous disease of worldwide distribution caused by gram-positive obligate parasites that are most closely related to bacteria. Illustrated here is the most common, cervicofacial form of the disease. Deep to this superficial neck mass is a focus of actinomycosis. The purulent discharge from the underlying sinus contains yellowish particles, so-called sulfur granules. These granules are colonies of the causative agent, which is usually *Actinomyces israelii*. Diagnosis is made by culture of the organism on anaerobic media, and the treatment of choice is penicillin.

Figure 54

Figure 55

Erythrasma This is a fairly common condition that is occasionally seen during childhood and increases in frequency with age. Lesions occur in the axillae, groin, and toewebs. The causative organism is a diphtheroid, *Corynebacterium minutissimum*. Involvement in the axilla, as seen in Fig. 54, appears as a brown-to-red well-demarcated plaque. Maceration and scaling between the toes (Fig. 55) is another clinical presentation. A characteristic of the lesion is that it fluoresces coral-red under the Wood's light (3650 Å), because the causative organism produces porphyrins in the stratum corneum. Erythrasma is exceedingly superficial but can become extensive. A 10-day course of oral erythromycin, 250 mg four times a day, is the treatment of choice.

4

Spirochetal, Protozoal, and Mycobacterial Diseases

Figure 56

Figure 57

Congenital syphilis In utero infection by the spirochete *Treponema pallidum* can occur after the sixteenth week of gestation. Intrauterine disease, especially during early pregnancy, may result in spontaneous abortion or in a severely affected infant. Severe disease that is present at birth presents with hepatosplenomegaly, ascites, meningoencephalitis, and severe anemia. Osteochondritis is the most characteristic bone change. The cutaneous findings in severe congenital syphilis include bullae, pustules, macules, and papules. Fis-

suring and peeling of the skin are also characteristic. The palms, soles, and periorificial skin are sites of predilection. Syphilitic rhinitis, with a copious and bloody nasal discharge, is an associated finding. If infection occurs late in pregnancy, signs and symptoms may be delayed for several weeks. In these cases, diagnosis is usually made on the basis of a positive syphilis serology in mother and infant. If allowed to progress, rhinitis, cutaneous macules, and mucous patches may be the presenting signs.

Figure 58

Figure 59

Acquired syphilis Unlike congenital syphilis, acquired syphilis in infants, children, and adolescents follows the classic course of syphilis in adults. Such an infection in a child should be assumed to be the result of sexual abuse. The first event in the development of syphilis is a dark-field positive chancre at the portal of entry of the treponeme. Shortly thereafter, serologic tests for syphilis become positive. Secondary syphilis usually develops 6 to 8 weeks after the appearance of the chancre. Malaise, low-grade fever, myal-

gias, and lymphadenopathy are accompanied by a wide variety of cutaneous manifestations. The lesions illustrated in Fig. 58 are condylomata lata on the genitalia. Note the moist papules and plaques. Figure 59 shows the most consistent form of skin disease in secondary syphilis. It consists of copper-colored papulosquamous lesions, most commonly on the palms and soles. Other cutaneous manifestations of secondary syphilis include papular lesions, pustules, nodules, plaques, and mucous patches.

Figure 60

Figure 61

Erythema chronicum migrans (Lyme disease) Lyme disease is caused by the spirochete *Borrelia burgdorferi* and is transmitted by the pinhead-sized Ixodid ticks. The illness is endemic in large areas of the continental United States. The early cutaneous manifestation, termed *erythema chronicum migrans,* is pictured here. It consists of an expanding annular lesion around the original tick bite. Satellite areas of involvement may also be present. Pruritus or burning may be present at the site of the lesion, and the rash may be accompanied by fever, malaise, and regional lymphadenopathy. The systemic manifestations of Lyme disease include neurologic dysfunction (e.g., Bell's palsy), cardiac conduction abnormalities, and arthritis. Early antibiotic therapy for the typical skin lesion will often prevent the development of the more serious and long-lasting systemic illness. Serologic testing is of some value in diagnosis, but may be negative early on, especially in the absence of neurologic or joint symptoms.

Figure 62

Figure 63

Yaws This is a nonvenereal treponematosis that is caused by *Treponema pertenue.* It is endemic in areas of Central and South America, Africa, and southeast Asia. The disease is acquired by physical contact, and the majority of cases occur during childhood. An ulceration occurs at the site of the primary inoculation. Secondary lesions are cutaneous nodules or moist or hyperkeratotic plaques; they appear within several weeks and resolve spontaneously. Recurrence of the latent disease, with gummata of the skin and bones, may occur many years later.

Amebiasis cutis *Entamoeba histolytica,* the cause of intestinal and cutaneous amebiasis, attains the skin from the intestinal infestation. Discharging from the ulcerous process in the lower part of the gut, viable amebas contaminate and may infect the perianal region especially. When the infection is seen in an active state, the process is a continually creeping, painful ulceration that has little tendency to heal spontaneously. When healed, the clinical appearance is a scar, as pictured.

Figure 64

Figure 65

Lepromatous leprosy   Leprosy, or Hansen's disease, is a chronic multisystem disease that is caused by *Mycobacterium leprae*, an acid-fast bacillus. The highest incidence of the disease is in areas of South America, Africa, and Asia. It is not rare in children. The clinical manifestations of this illness depend on the host response to infection. At one end of the spectrum is lepromatous leprosy (LL), which represents a diminished host response to the leprosy bacillus. Cutaneous lesions in this form of the disease vary. Macular lesions are

symmetrically distributed, hypopigmented, and erythematous patches. When widespread involvement occurs, the lesions may be difficult to differentiate from normal skin. The lesions pictured here are more infiltrative. Nodular lesions of the earlobe, as illustrated in Fig. 64, are particularly common in lepromatous leprosy. Annular plaques and papules (Fig. 65) may also be present. Lepromatous leprosy is the form most likely to cause widespread nerve damage and ocular disease.

Figure 66

Figure 67

Tuberculoid leprosy   Patients with tuberculoid leprosy (classification TT) are those who have the strongest immune response to chronic infection. The cutaneous lesions are typically sharply demarcated plaques with a firm raised border. Varying degrees of erythema, hypopigmentation, and anesthesia may be present. Note the large sharply demarcated areas of decreased pigmentation in Fig. 66, and the raised border of the lesion in Fig. 67. In early disease, the loss of sensation and normal sweating in involved areas may be

difficult to detect, and the lesions can easily be confused with vitiligo and pityriasis alba. Tuberculoid leprosy tends to remain a localized disease, and spontaneous resolution may occur. Nerve damage tends to be limited to one or two nerves. The treatment of all forms of leprosy is now complicated by the appearance of dapsone resistance. Combinations of rifampicin, clofazimine, and dapsone are now required in many cases.

Figure 68

Figure 69

Dimorphous leprosy   The terms *borderline* or *dimorphous* leprosy are used to refer to patients whose disease shows features of both the lepromatous and tuberculoid forms. Patients with dimorphous leprosy (classified as BL, BB, or BT) have varied skin lesions, including the plaques and annular lesions that are illustrated in Figs. 68 and 69. They often suffer widespread and rapidly progressive nerve damage. Knowledge of the proper treatment of leprosy must include an understanding of the acute exacerbations that may

accompany therapy. Treatment of nonlepromatous leprosy with antibiotics may induce erythema and edema of the skin lesions, accompanied by rapid damage to the peripheral nerves (Type I reaction). Type II reaction, also termed *erythema nodosum leprosum*, is most common in patients with lepromatous leprosy. It consists of painful dermal nodules accompanied by ocular disease, peripheral neuropathies, and a wide variety of constitutional symptoms.

Figure 70

Figure 71

Histopathology of lepromatous leprosy   Exposure to and contact with *Mycobacterium leprae, Mycobacterium tuberculosis,* and other microorganisms of the genus do not produce overt or detectable disease in all, not even in most, individuals. Only a few develop clinical disease. In the matter of leprosy, there are two polar types of overt disease, namely, lepromatous and tuberculoid leprosy. In the tuberculoid form, organisms are sparse and the histologic response to them is granulomatous in a manner similar to that seen in sarcoidosis

and some forms of tuberculosis. In the lepromatous form, here illustrated, organisms are abundant, and the histologic response is characteristically in the form of sheets of histiocytes that are laden with lepra bacilli and that have foamy, vacuolated cytoplasm. Typically a zone of uninvolved connective tissue, well shown in the photomicrograph (Fig. 70), separates the epidermis from the disease process in the dermis. Lepra bacilli are readily revealed by any method of staining for acid-fast bacilli (Fig. 71).

Figure 72

Figure 73

Primary complex of tuberculosis in the skin A child with an area of injury to the skin may develop a primary complex in that location when exposed to someone with active tuberculosis. After an incubation period of 1–3 weeks, a red papule develops and evolves into a nodule or plaque with ulceration. The tuberculous ulcer is accompanied by regional lymphadenopathy. This form of cutaneous tuberculosis is a self-limited disease, and slow healing with scar formation occurs. A stage in this process is shown.

Lupus vulgaris This is a progressive form of cutaneous tuberculosis that results from the hematogenous spread of *Mycobacterium tuberculosis*. It is seen in patients who are very sensitive to the organism. Favored locations are the central face, earlobes, and other parts of the head and neck. The lesions may be papules, nodules, or plaques, and the color is often described as "apple jelly." Older lesions (Fig. 73) are brownish, annular plaques; the area of central clearing represents an attempt at healing.

Figure 74

Figure 75

Tuberculosis cutis colliquativa (scrofuloderma) This type of cutaneous tuberculosis results from the extension of infection from an underlying location to the skin. The original site of involvement may be a joint, bone, or visceral organ, but most commonly it is a lymph node. Illustrated here is a case of tuberculous cervical lymphadenitis, with the channelling of sinuses to the skin surface. This form of cutaneous infection by *M. tuberculosis* is particularly common in children.

Tuberculosis cutis verrucosa This form of cutaneous tuberculosis results form exogenous reinfection of an already tuberculin-sensitive individual. When the lesions are located on the hands or feet, they tend to develop a distinctly verrucous surface, beneath which is inflammation. This representation is characteristic. There is most likely a history of prior injury to the foot.

Figure 76

Figure 77

Lichen scrofulosorum This title describes a condition that consists of grouped lichenoid papules on the trunk. It occurs in children who have active tuberculosis in other locations. The individual lesions are flat-topped, follicular papules and are either erythematous or flesh colored. The condition is asymptomatic and follows a benign course to spontaneous resolution.

Papulonecrotic tuberculid Clinically this condition is highly stereotypic. It consists of dusky, red, matchhead- to pea-sized, sterile papules that arise in symmetrical crops on the extensor aspects of the extremities, usually on the elbows and knees. Occasionally the buttocks are also involved. The condition is asymptomatic and heals spontaneously with varioliform scars.

Figure 78

Figure 79

Histopathology of tuberculosis cutis Cutaneous tuberculosis may be divided into two categories, one in which the response is to living organisms present in tissue and another in which the response is to particulate or soluble products of organisms hematogenously disseminated from an occult focus of living organisms. The latter responses are commonly referred to as tuberculids. The histopathology of response to living organisms and their products depends on immunologic developments. When the skin becomes the portal of entry of tubercle bacilli, the early response is banal inflammation, and the later response is granulomatous with central necrosis (Fig. 78). Thereafter, responses to tubercle bacilli, endogenously disseminated or exogenously reacquired, are almost instantly granulomatous in the form of collections of epithelioid and giant cells seated in a sea of lymphocytes and with little or no necrosis (caseation). This is the typical picture of lupus vulgaris (Fig. 79).

Figure 80

Figure 81

Infection with atypical mycobacteria   There are a number of cutaneous infections that are caused by mycobacteria other than *M. tuberculosis* or *M. leprae*. Illustrated here is infection by *Mycobacterium marinum*. This organism is known to contaminate fish tanks and swimming pools, and the cutaneous infection is sometimes termed *swimming pool granuloma*. In fact, the case in Fig. 80 was traced to a fish tank, and that in Fig. 81 to a swimming pool. The lesions usually appear at a point of trauma, and the hands, feet, elbows, and knees are particularly common locations. After an incubation period of 2 to 6 weeks, the lesions evolve from small papules into single or grouped violaceous nodules. Satellite lesions may be present. Biopsy of a mature lesion reveals a caseating granuloma, and acid-fast organisms within histiocytes can sometimes be identified. Diagnosis can also be made by culture of biopsied material.

Figure 82

Figure 83

Histopathology of infection with atypical mycobacteria There are numerous mycobacteria that resemble *Mycobacterium tuberculosis* and have similar, though less virulent, pathogenicity. *Mycobacterium marinum* is one such organism. The reaction that results depends again upon complex immunologic developments. The usual clinical picture is a verrucous process of which the histopathology is, as shown, epidermal hyperplasia, intraepidermal abscess formation, and tuberculoid inflammatory process with giant cells in the dermis.

Infection with atypical mycobacteria   This illustration is another instance of granulomatous process caused by a mycobacterium other than that of tuberculosis. In this case, the organism was *Mycobacterium intracellulare*. The lesion resembles that of tuberculosis cutis colliquativa. The causative organism was cultured from the discharge that issued from sinuses emerging from infected lymph nodes. The patient was positive in reaction to conventional tuberculin and to tuberculins derived from so-called atypical mycobacteria.

Figure 84

Figure 85

Leishmaniasis The cutaneous form of leishmaniasis is caused by a protozoan (*Leishmania tropica*) that is transmitted by the bite of a sandfly (of the genus *Phlebotomus*) in certain endemic regions (the Middle East, China, Africa, India, the Soviet Union). The primary process in the skin starts as a macule of erythema, evolves into a papule (Fig. 84), and then into a granulomatous or ulcerous process (Fig. 85). The lesion takes up to 1 year to heal spontaneously in the form of a vacciniform scar. Systemic leishmaniasis (kala-azar) is caused by the related protozoan *Leishmania donovani*. This form is characterized by fever, anemia, leukopenia, emaciation, and severe hepatosplenomegaly. The skin develops a grayish pigmentation, usually on the face. Finally, mucocutaneous leishmaniasis is caused by *Leishmania braziliensis*, is characterized by destructive mucosal lesions, and is endemic in some areas of Latin America.

5

Viral and Rickettsial Diseases

Figure 86

Figure 87

Molluscum contagiosum This condition is a benign viral infection which appears as crops of discrete, slightly umbilicated, flesh-colored or shiny papules. It is extremely common among children and may be seen in several children within a family. The lesions may become inflamed if traumatized or infected and sometimes become inflamed spontaneously as they resolve. Rarely is there only a solitary lesion; most commonly there are less than 20. However, the total number is sometimes in the hundreds. The lesions tend to be grouped, and the average size of a lesion is 2–3 mm in diameter and

height. The trunk, face, and genitalia are the most common sites of infection. Pruritus is an occasional symptom and may be the impetus for inoculating the viral infection from one area of the skin to another. Molluscum contagiosum is self-limited, but treatment is often required out of concern for appearance. Treatment should be individualized to the age and extent of involvement in each patient. Destruction of lesions with a sharp curette is the preferred mode in a cooperative child with limited disease. The child with numerous lesions poses a particular therapeutic challenge.

Figure 88

Figure 89

Molluscum contagiosum Occasionally, a lesion of molluscum contagiosum may grow to as large as 3 cm in diameter. Two such "giant mollusca" are pictured here. The diagnosis is usually suggested by the presence of more typical, smaller lesions on adjacent or distant skin surfaces. Treatment is again by surgical removal when possible. Local anesthesia would be a feasible and a kind thing to administer in such a case.

Histopathology of molluscum contagiosum Molluscum contagiosum is a viral disease which takes the form of small tumors in which the virus can be visualized within a characteristic histopathologic picture. In the upper layers of epidermal cells, viral inclusions are seen as collections known as *molluscum bodies* when they have developed to occupy the entire cytoplasmic space of those cells in the form of amphophilic or slightly basophilic structures. This phenomenon is most clearly seen in and about the stratum granulosum.

Figure 90

Figure 91

Verruca vulgaris The common wart is a benign growth caused by localized infection with one of the many types of human papillomavirus. These small DNA viruses are part of the papova group. Warts are especially common among children and adolescents and may occur on any mucocutaneous surface. The hands are a particularly frequent location. The typical wart is a rough-surfaced nodule that may be either lighter or darker than the surrounding skin. Lesions involving the proximal and lateral nail folds are pictured in

Fig. 90; Fig. 91 shows numerous verrucae on the palmar surface. Treatment must be individualized to the age and cooperative abilities of the patient, and to the size and location of the wart. For some lesions, the simplest and most effective approach is treatment by desiccation and curettage. In other cases, cryotherapy or treatment with a salicylic acid preparation is preferable. The gentler forms of treatment are particularly good for periungual warts. In those areas, surgery may cause scarring of the nail matrix and nail dystrophy.

Figure 92

Figure 93

Verruca plantaris Plantar warts appear as flat areas of firm hyperkeratosis on the soles of the feet. Lesions that occur at points of pressure may be associated with severe pain on walking. Figure 92 illustrates a solitary plantar wart. Note the obliteration of skin markings, which does not occur in a callus. The lesions in Fig. 93 are numerous and mosaic. Treatment of plantar warts requires perseverance on the part of both patient and physician. Attempts at a rapid cure may

result in scarring. One practical method involves the daily application of salicylic acid plasters or liquid salicylic acid preparations, along with repeated paring of the necrotic surface of the wart. The success of this routine may be hastened by gentle cryotherapy. Lesions that are small and in non-weight bearing areas may be removed by curettage without electrocautery.

Figure 94

Verruca filiformis The surfaces of common warts are influenced by their positions on the body and by what goes on there. In general they are rough of surface. On hands, the surfaces of warts are domed from wear and tear so that troughs and crests are shallow; on soles, they are flat and smooth from the weight of the body; but where they are undisturbed, common warts tend to grow with fimbria or finger-like projections. They are then called *filiform* or *digitate*. The face and scalp are the most common sites where warts grow in this fashion.

Figure 95

Condyloma acuminatum Warts with this "cauliflower" appearance on the labia, penis, or around the rectum are termed *condylomata acuminata*. The presence of lesions of this type in a child should prompt the physician to consider the possibility of sexual abuse, although the true incidence of this association is not known. In some cases, condylomata acuminata may be the result of innocent contact with another infected individual, or perinatal transmission from a mother with cervical or vaginal lesions. Brief application of podophyllum resin is the preferred treatment.

Figure 96

Verruca plana Plane, or flat, warts may be caused by several types of the human papillomavirus. They are common in children. The lesions are slightly raised, flesh-colored papules, usually 2–4 mm in diameter. The face and hands are the most frequent location for these multiple small warts. The lesions may be discrete or confluent, and a linear array of flat warts may result from autoinoculation in a scratch. Gentle freezing or chemical destruction are the treatments of choice.

Figure 97

Epidermodysplasia verruciformis This rare familial disease usually has its onset during childhood. Patients develop numerous flat warts, initially involving the face and upper trunk. A number of human papillomavirus types have been implicated. As the lesions tend towards confluence, they may mimic the appearance of tinea versicolor. Most patients with epidermodysplasia verruciformis have depressed cell-mediated immunity. They are also at risk for squamous cell carcinomas, which generally arise on sun-exposed skin.

Figure 98

Neonatal herpes simplex Neonatal herpes simplex infection is acquired during passage through an infected birth canal. The cutaneous involvement may be as extensive as pictured here, or it may be subtle. The scalp is the most common site for the typical clustered vesicles. Because of the very high frequency of concurrent disseminated disease, cutaneous herpes simplex in the newborn must be considered a pediatric emergency. Early treatment with an intravenous antiviral agent offers the infant the best possibility of survival.

Figure 99

Herpetic whitlow Herpes simplex infection of the distal phalanx may occur in infants and young children. The first episode may accompany herpetic gingivostomatitis. Herpetic whitlow presents with pain or paresthesia and with erythema and vesiculation. The original infection is occasionally mis-diagnosed as a bacterial paronychia. Subsequent recurrences of lesions in the same site, which occur in about 20 percent of patients, will lead the practitioner to the correct diagnosis.

Figure 100

Herpes progenitalis Herpes simplex infection in the genital region is a sexually transmitted disease. It is not uncommon in the sexually active adolescent, as pictured here. In the young child, genital herpes simplex should create a high index of suspicion for sexual abuse. This figure illustrates the multiple painful erosions which may occur in primary infection. Regional lymphadenopathy and fever may also be present. Recurrences of genital herpes are very common but are generally much milder both in extent and duration than the primary disease.

Figure 101

Herpes simplex, recurrent Here illustrated is a severe case of recurrent herpes simplex on the eyelids, cheek, and nose. Without a clear history of recurrence, herpes zoster would enter into the differential diagnosis. Repeated corneal ulcer-ation, with scarring, may lead to visual impairment. Herpes simplex keratitis has become the major cause of infectious blindness in the United States.

Figure 102

Figure 103

Herpes simplex, recurrent (cont.) Following an episode of primary herpes simplex, the virus may remain dormant within a nerve ganglion. A number of triggering factors, including febrile illness, emotional or physical stress, excessive sun exposure, and trauma, may cause the virus to replicate and spread to the skin surface. The typical "fever blister" or "cold sore" is a recurrent herpes simplex infection on the lip or vermillion border. Genital herpes simplex infection is

also, more often than not, characterized by periodic recurrence. Patients with recurrent disease will often experience prodromal pain or paresthesia in the involved area. Most episodes last from 7 to 10 days. Represented here are lesions on the face (Fig. 102) and on the knee (Fig. 103). The latter is a less common location, serving to illustrate that recurrent herpes simplex may occur on any area of the skin.

Figure 104

Figure 105

Eczema herpeticum (Kaposi's varicelliform eruption) Disseminated cutaneous herpes simplex infection is a serious complication of atopic dermatitis. It may also occasionally occur in individuals with other dermatological disorders. Patients rapidly develop numerous umbilicated vesicles in the areas of eczematous involvement. Children with eczema herpeticum often become seriously ill with high fever. Bacterial superinfection and sepsis can be a complication, and the disease is occasionally fatal. The patients pictured here

developed involvement of the entire skin surface. The lesions in Fig. 105 are typical umbilicated vesicles; those in Fig. 104 are equally extensive and are beginning to crust. Skillful and attentive supportive treatment is required in order to maintain fluid and electrolyte balance and prevent superinfection. Treatment with intravenous acyclovir seems to hasten clinical improvement and is often recommended for children with extensive or rapidly increasing involvement.

Figure 106

Figure 107

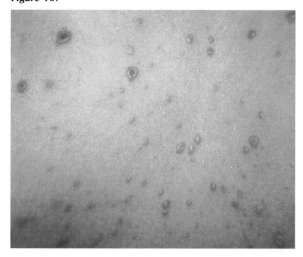

Varicella Chickenpox is caused by a virus of the herpes group. The disease is highly contagious and is spread by droplet or direct contact. The incubation period for chickenpox ranges from 11 to 21 days. Prodromal symptoms consist of low-grade fever, headache, anorexia, and malaise. On the following day, the characteristic rash begins to appear. The lesions evolve from erythematous macules to form small papules. Quickly, a clear vesicle arises on this erythematous base. The classic lesion of chickenpox has been poetically described as a "dewdrop on a rose petal." Over the next several days, the vesicles rupture and then crust. The rash begins on the chest and back, and spreads centrifugally to involve the face, scalp, and extremities. New lesions of chickenpox arise in crops over a period of several days. Since crops of macules-papules-vesicles-crusts are successive and overlapping, one sees lesions at all stages of development in given locations. Itching is a symptom and may be severe.

Figure 108

Figure 109

Varicella Lesions on the oral mucous membranes, which are common, are pictured in Fig. 109. They are most common on the palate and quickly evolve into small, superficial erosions. Fig. 108 depicts a case of chickenpox of unusual severity. The lesions tend to be large blisters and to become hemorrhagic. Cases of this type are more likely to occur in children with reticuloendothelial malignancies, with immunologic defects, or in those under immunosuppressive or prolonged adrenocorticosteroid therapy. Complications of chickenpox in these children may include varicella pneumonia, myocarditis, and hepatitis. There are also a number of complications of chickenpox in the child who was previously healthy. Secondary bacterial infection of the skin lesions is by far the most common. Other, less frequent, sequelae include thrombocytopenia, purpura fulminans, and postinfectious encephalitis. Finally, a significant number of cases of Reye syndrome occur after chickenpox, and aspirin should therefore not be used as an antipyretic.

Figure 110

Congenital varicella syndrome   On rare occasions, the infants of mothers who develop chickenpox during the first trimester of pregnancy are born with congenital defects. The congenital varicella syndrome is characterized by asymmetrical arm or leg lengths, ocular abnormalities, microcephaly, and intra-uterine growth retardation. Cutaneous scarring in a derma-tomal distribution is particularly characteristic of the con-stellation of birth defects caused by the varicella-zoster virus.

Figure 111

Neonatal varicella   Maternal chickenpox in the several days before or after the birth of a child may lead to a significant health risk for the infant. The newborn who is exposed to varicella without the benefit of transplacental maternal anti-body may go on to develop severe, disseminated infection with pulmonary and hepatic involvement. This disease may sometimes be fatal. Pictured here is a newborn with numerous typical chickenpox lesions over the face. The hemorrhagic lesions that may be part of neonatal varicella are not present in this child.

Figure 112

Figure 113

Herpes zoster   Herpes zoster, or shingles, is an acute erup-tion characterized by vesicles and small bullae. Lesions are usually unilateral and confined to a single dermatome. The cause of herpes zoster is the varicella-zoster virus. After an initial episode of chickenpox, the virus lies dormant in the dorsal root or cranial nerve ganglia. Reactivation of the virus, usually years later, leads to the typical eruption. Herpes zoster is a relatively rare disease in children and is seen more frequently in those young people who had had chickenpox at a very early age. Localized pain may precede the onset of the rash, but postherpetic neuralgia is unusual in childhood. Children with lesions around the eye or on the tip of the nose may have involvement of the nasociliary nerve and should be observed carefully for ocular involvement.

Figure 114

Figure 115

Generalized herpes zoster The child with herpes zoster may, in the normal course of the illness, develop several chickenpox-like lesions outside of the involved dermatome. However, rapid and widespread evolution of such lesions—generalized herpes zoster—is a problem of greater concern. Hematogenous spread of the viral infection in this fashion may be an indication of an underlying immune deficiency.

Histopathology of varicella and herpes zoster Chickenpox and shingles are caused by the same virus, one of the two in the herpes group that are pathogenic to man. Both viruses of the group produce intraepidermal blisters that are different from those caused by pox viruses. Distinctive features are enlargement of epithelial cells, margination of chromatin, frequent multinucleation, and sometimes nuclear atypia. In varicella and herpes zoster, inflammatory infiltrates are rare; the opposite is true in herpes simplex.

Figure 116

Figure 117

Hand-foot-mouth disease This common and benign viral disease of childhood is usually caused by the A16 strain of coxsackievirus, although other strains of the same virus have been implicated. It most often occurs in late summer and early fall. The prodrome consists of low-grade fever and malaise. Shortly thereafter, vesicular lesions arise on the soft palate (Fig. 116), tongue, buccal mucosa, and uvula. The lips are usually spared. Occasionally, these lesions may be painful and cause some difficulty in eating. The cutaneous lesions develop 1 or 2 days subsequent to those in the mouth. They

consist of asymptomatic round or oval vesiculopustules that evolve into superficial erosions. The edges of the palms and soles are a favored location (Fig. 117). The dorsae of the hands and feet may also be involved. There is sometimes an accompanying macular and papular eruption on the buttocks. The eruption lasts from 7 to 10 days, and no therapy is required. Although culture of the virus is possible, the diagnosis of hand-foot-mouth disease is usually made on clinical grounds.

Figure 118

Figure 119

Complications of vaccinia The worldwide eradication of smallpox has eliminated the need for vaccination with the modified cowpox virus. Over the many years that this medical practice was necessary, a number of benign and some more serious dermatologic complications were observed. The sequelae of smallpox vaccination are as follows: 3–4 days after inoculation, there develops an area of erythema and edema at the injection site (usually an arm or thigh); this rapidly evolves into edema, vesiculation, ulceration, crusting, and scar formation over a period of about 3 weeks. For most children, fever, malaise, and local discomfort are the major side effects. The complications of a severe local reaction (Fig. 118), and of a generalized eruption (Figs. 118, 119), are illustrated here.

Figure 120

Figure 121

Complications of vaccinia Still another complication of premeditated induction of vaccinia may be very serious, namely, accidental autoinoculation on an undesirable site while the primary pock is in progress. Autoinoculation then results in a new lesion that begins in a day (a reaction time) and rapidly repeats the whole process. The seriousness of such accidents lies in the site: on the face, particularly around the eyes, blindness, and elsewhere on exposed skin, cosmetic defects, are serious consequences.

Eczema vaccinatum Disseminated vaccinia is the most dreaded complication of smallpox vaccination. Like eczema herpeticum, eczema vaccinatum occurs in children with underlying eczematous disorders. It is more serious because of the severity of the acute illness, the tendency toward scarring, and a higher incidence of mortality. The illustration suggests that the scarring from eczema vaccinatum can be disfiguring.

Figure 122

Figure 123

Echovirus disease A wide variety of enteroviruses of the echovirus and coxsackievirus groups are responsible for similar systemic illnesses and cutaneous eruptions. These illnesses are all most common in the late summer or early fall. In the case of echovirus, there is an incubation period of 3–7 days, followed by the sudden onset of fever and myalgia. Some combination of abdominal pain, vomiting, pharyngitis, and cervical adenopathy may also be present. Occasionally, nuchal rigidity may indicate the presence of aseptic meningitis. The eruption begins to develop on the face (Fig. 122), and, shortly, within hours, generalization to the trunk (Fig. 123) and limbs occurs. The lesions, which are erythematous, papular, and rubelliform, persist for about 3–5 days, and then recede. Occasionally, the virus can be recovered from throat, urine, or stool. There is no specific treatment, and little more than simple supportive therapy is required until spontaneous recovery takes place.

Figure 124

Figure 125

Exanthem subitum (Roseola) Roseola is a common childhood illness which is now known to be caused by human herpesvirus 6. Most cases occur during the first year of life. The disease is characterized by 3–5 days of high fever accompanied by minimal constitutional symptoms. Pharyngitis, periorbital edema, and cervical adenopathy may be present, and febrile convulsions sometimes occur. The disappearance of the fever is accompanied by the onset of rash. The typical eruption is macular and papular, and concentrated on the neck and trunk. The eruption clears in hours, or at most a day or two.

Papular acrodermatitis of childhood (Gianotti-Crosti syndrome) This condition is characterized by the eruption of firm erythematous papules on the extremities, cheeks, and buttocks. The papulonodular lesions may become confluent in some areas. This disease was originally described in children with anicteric hepatitis B infection. Since that time, Gianotti-Crosti syndrome has been found to occur in association with coxsackie, parainfluenza, and Epstein-Barr virus infection. Other causes are poliovirus, vaccinia, β-hemolytic streptococcus, and bacille Calmette-Guérin (BCG).

Figure 126

Cytomegalic inclusion disease   Congenital infection with cytomegalovirus, a DNA virus of the herpes group, results in disease of varying severity. Whereas some neonates are completely asymptomatic, severely affected infants display intrauterine growth retardation, microcephaly, and hepatosplenomegaly. The cutaneous manifestations, pictured here, are petechiae and purpura. The "blueberry muffin" spots are an indication of extramedullary hematopoiesis. Culture of the virus from urine is the most specific means of diagnosis.

Figure 127

Congenital rubella   In utero infection by the rubella virus during the first 20 weeks of gestation may result in severe, multisystem involvement and a variety of developmental defects. Illustrated here are the dark-blue-to-purple "blueberry muffin" lesions in the severely affected neonate. They are a sign of extramedullary hematopoiesis. Thrombocytopenic purpura is an additional cutaneous manifestation. Congenital cataracts, deafness, and cardiac malformations form a classic triad in infants with the severe intrauterine infection.

Figure 128

Rubella   This common viral disease affects both children and young adults. A mild prodrome consists of headache, coryza, and low-grade fever. The rash itself varies enormously in its course and duration. Most typically, it begins on the face and neck and spreads to the trunk and extremities, as pictured here, over 1–2 days. The lesions are small pink macules and maculopapules, which rapidly coalesce and then fade. The rash is so evanescent that it may begin to disappear on the face before developing on the trunk and extremities. Petechiae

Figure 129

on the soft palate, termed *Forchheimer's sign,* are present in some patients (Fig. 129). Systemic illness is generally mild. Enlargement of suboccipital and posterior auricular lymph nodes is a characteristic physical finding. The most serious aspect of rubella is the severe developmental defects which may result from intrauterine infection during the first trimester. Routine childhood immunization has resulted in fewer epidemics and therefore in a lower incidence of viral exposure to pregnant women.

Figure 130

Figure 131

Measles Rubeola, or measles, is a systemic illness caused by an RNA paramyxovirus. The incidence of this previously common childhood disease has decreased markedly since the advent of an effective vaccine, but measles has by no means been eradicated. After an incubation period of 1–2 weeks, the infected child develops fever, conjunctivitis, photophobia, and a distinctive brassy or barking cough. Frequently, the fever and constitutional symptoms are severe. A day or two after onset of these constitutional signs and symptoms, the

enanthem (Koplik's spots) appears as bright red puncta with central blue-white flecks on the buccal mucosa opposite the second molars (Fig. 130). The characteristic rash is maculo-papular and erythematous. It begins on the forehead and behind the ears and spreads to the face (Fig. 131), neck, trunk, and extremities. The rash disappears in the same sequence, sometimes leaving areas of fine desquamation. The duration of the entire illness is usually 5–7 days.

Figure 132

Figure 133

Measles This picture shows the "measly" appearance of a child who clearly feels miserable. The disease is brief and self-limited for most children, and the treatment is entirely supportive. The incidence of complications is higher, how-ever, than in the other childhood exanthems. Otitis media is the most common. Serious complications include broncho-pneumonia and encephalitis, which may cause permanent neurologic damage. Subacute sclerosing panencephalitis is a late sequela of measles.

Atypical measles Children who received the "killed" mea-sles vaccine, available during the mid-1960s, may develop "atypical measles" upon exposure to the virus as young adults. This disease is characterized by high fever and severe respiratory symptoms. The accompanying rash is frequently compared to that of Rocky Mountain spotted fever (Figs. 136 and 137). The exanthem, which typically begins on the hands and feet, may be macular, vesicular, or purpuric. Children who receive the live attenuated measles vaccine, which is currently in use, are not susceptible to atypical measles.

Figure 134

Figure 135

Rickettsialpox This self-limited febrile illness is caused by *Rickettsia akari*. It is transmitted to man by a mite that is an obligatory parasite of the common house mouse. One to two weeks after exposure, a nodule develops at the point of entry of a parasitized mite. The nodule becomes vesicular and then crusted with a black eschar (the pock, seen well developed on the neck in Fig. 134). Regional lymphadenopathy is usually present. Within several days, the patient develops intermittent

fever, photophobia, headache, myalgia, and lassitude. Two or three days later, a generalized exanthem, consisting of discrete macules that quickly become papular, appears (Fig. 135). Firm vesiculopustules arise atop the papules, and these subsequently form crusts. The eruption lasts 1–2 weeks. Unlike Rocky Mountain spotted fever, rickettsialpox shows a negative Weil-Felix reaction.

Figure 136

Figure 137

Rocky Mountain spotted fever This disease is caused by *Rickettsia rickettsii* and is transmitted by a number of different ticks. Despite its geographical title, Rocky Mountain spotted fever is present in many locations throughout the United States and the entire Western Hemisphere. After infection by tick bite, there is an incubation period of 2–14 days. The abrupt onset of the disease includes severe headache, fever, chills, arthralgia, and myalgia. After 2–3 days of these constitutional symptoms, erythematous macules erupt on the wrists, hands, forearms, legs, and ankles (Figs. 136, 137).

Lesions then spread to the palms and soles and the trunk. The macules originally blanch with pressure but soon become purpuric and even necrotic. The disease causes a severe vasculitis, and complications include disseminated intravascular coagulation, hemorrhage into the gastrointestinal and urinary tracts, and cardiovascular collapse. The Weil-Felix test is positive, but the disease must be treated immediately upon clinical suspicion. The high fatality rate is markedly reduced by prompt antibiotic therapy.

Figure 138

Figure 139

Erythema infectiosum (fifth disease)   Erythema infectiosum is a mild childhood disease which is now known to be caused by human parvovirus B19. This condition develops after a mean incubation period of 14 days. There are few if any prodromal symptoms. The rash evolves in three clinical stages. The first stage is characterized by the abrupt appearance of a bright red malar blush.. The appearance is so startling that it has been given the suggestive description of "slapped cheeks" (Fig. 138). During the second stage, the facial rash begins to fade, and a maculopapular, urticarial, or morbilliform exanthem develops on the extremities and trunk. Pruritus may be present. As portions of this rash fade over a period of several days, a reticular pattern emerges, mainly on the extremities, which gives the arms and legs a marbled appearance (Fig. 139). This reticular eruption, which is the third stage of the disease, may last only 1 week, or it may last continuously or by relapses for as long as 8 weeks. Exercise and variations in temperature may make the rash appear more or less prominent. No treatment is required.

Fungal Infections

Figure 140

Figure 141

Tinea capitis Fungal infections of the scalp are extremely common in children. The diagnosis of tinea capitis should be entertained in any child in whom patches of incomplete alopecia crusting or scaling are found in the scalp. In previous decades, *Microsporum canis* and *M. audouinii* were the most common pathogenic fungi infecting the scalp. The latter frequently causes a discrete, grayish patch of hair loss (Fig. 141) In most parts of the United States and in many other parts of the world, *Trichophyton tonsurans* is now the

predominant organism causing tinea capitis. In some children, this dermatophyte causes discrete and dramatic areas of hair loss studded by the stubs of broken hairs, the so-called black dot ringworm (Fig. 140). In others, there are only small and unimpressive patches of ''seborrheic'' scale with minimal hair loss, or groups of small pustules. Because *T. tonsurans* does not fluoresce, the Wood's light is no longer of use in most cases. However, diagnosis can be confirmed by the use of either KOH preparation or fungal culture.

Figure 142

Figure 143

Tinea capitis Pictured here is an inflammatory response to infection with *Trichophyton tonsurans*. Children whose scalps are infected with this dermatophyte may also develop regional lymphadenopathy or a fine papular eruption which spreads from the face and neck to other skin surfaces (the id reaction). Attempts to treat tinea capitis with topical antifungals alone are doomed to failure. Oral griseofulvin is the most effective form of therapy. The use of a selenium sulfide shampoo may be effective in preventing spread to classmates and siblings.

Kerion In some children, an exuberant inflammatory response to the infecting dermatophyte may occur. This boggy and tender mass is termed a *kerion*, a word that in Greek means a honeycomb, honey, or beeswax and is intended to describe the clinical appearance. Children with a kerion may also develop localized lymphadenopathy and fever. Misdiagnosis of a kerion as a bacterial infection of the scalp is an all too common pitfall. The proper treatment is oral griseofulvin. In some cases, a brief course of oral prednisone may minimize scarring.

Figure 144

Figure 145

Tinea corporis (ringworm) Superficial fungal infections of the skin are among the most common of all pediatric dermatoses. Infection at the sites pictured here may also be termed *tinea faciei*. Note the ring shape of the active periphery of the lesions in the infant in Fig. 144 and the more inflammatory process in the patient in Fig. 145. *Trichophyton tonsurans, T. rubrum,* and *T. mentagrophytes* are common pathogens. Cutaneous infection with zoophilic species, such as *Microsporum canis,* usually results from close contact with a household pet. On the body, fungi lodge in the stratum corneum and do not invade lanugo hairs. Therefore, topically applied antifungal agents, such as econazole, miconazole and clotrimazole, are effective therapy. Occasionally, a cutaneous fungal infection, particularly on the face, is misdiagnosed as atopic or contact dermatitis. The application of topical steroids to such a lesion will often cause dramatic worsening of the condition.

Figure 146

Figure 147

Tinea corporis (ringworm) The illustrations are of more superficial fungal infection of relatively hairless skin. The annular lesion in Fig. 146 resulted from infection with *Trichophyton tonsurans*. The numerous scaly rings in Fig. 147 are due to *Microsporum canis*. In the cases illustrated, clinical diagnosis of a superficial fungal infection is reasonably certain, and one may guess that the causative fungus is a microsporum or trichophyton. Definitive diagnosis depends on mycologic culture of the scale from a lesion. In cases of candidiasis, favus, and tinea imbricata (see Fig. 160), the causative organism can frequently and confidently be guessed correctly. In general one may say that *Microsporum canis, M. audouinii, Trichophyton tonsurans,* and *T. schoenleinii* can infect scalp and hairless skin; *T. rubrum* and *Candida albicans,* hairless skin and nails.

Figure 148

Tinea corporis (cont.) Here illustrated is superficial fungal infection of glabrous skin caused by *Microsporum gypseum.* The clinical appearance is somewhat different from the condition caused by other dermatophytes in that, while a round lesion, it is not a ring of active periphery around a relatively healed center. Still, the superficiality, the scaling, and the low-grade inflammatory reaction are typical of a fungous infection; it can be proved by culture of the causative fungus.

Figure 149

Tinea cruris The groins are common sites of acute and then enduring superficial fungal infection. *Epidermophyton floccosum, Trichophyton rubrum,* and *Candida albicans* are the commonest infecting fungi. In infants, *Candida albicans* is the usual pathogen; in older children and adults, all are common. Intertriginous spaces, such as groins, axillae, and digital webs, are particularly susceptible to fungal infection because the pH of these areas is less acid than elsewhere, temperature is higher, and humidity is greater.

Figure 150

Tinea pedis Superficial fungal infection of the feet is somewhat unique because of the location. Between the toes (most commonly the fourth and fifth), the condition appears as erythema, maceration, and scaling. It is attended by itching or vague discomfort. On the sole and the lateral aspects of the feet, scattered pustules and vesicles, with surrounding erythema and edema may occur (Fig. 150). More commonly, there is persistent dry scale in a "moccasin" distribution, with minimal inflammation (Fig. 151). The fungi that are commonly found are *Epidermophyton floccosum, Trichophy-*

Figure 151

ton mentagrophytes, Trichophyton rubrum, and *Candida albicans.* Fungal infections of the feet are rare in infants and young children, and scaling and erythema of the feet is more likely due to juvenile plantar dermatosis or contact dermatitis. Sweating, friction, and debris promote fungal infection. During early adolescence, there is a marked increase in the incidence of tinea pedis. For most patients, the use of topical antifungal therapy, along with the wearing of sandals and light cotton socks, is adequate therapy.

Figure 152

Figure 153

Onychomycosis Tinea unguium (fungal infection of the nails) is extremely uncommon during childhood. After puberty, its frequency increases with age. Usually, onychomycosis is associated with tinea pedis. Fungal culture of the nails is at times difficult but extremely important in confirming the diagnosis. Onychomycosis is the most difficult of the superficial fungal infections to treat because the nail plate is not penetrated by topically applied agents. Griseofulvin is only partially satisfactory. Usually, months of therapy are required for both fingernails and toenails. The relapse rate is very

high. Topical treatment with an imidazole solution is sometimes rewarding, especially if combined with mechanical removal of diseased nail and good local care. The illustrations show infection with dermatophytes. Note the distortion of nail plates in Fig. 152 and the onycholysis (separation of plates from nail beds) in Fig. 153. Infection by dermatophytes usually proceeds in a distal to proximal direction. Infection of nails by *Candida albicans* is different in that it is more acute (frequently purulent) and tends first to involve the lateral and proximal nail folds.

Figure 154

Figure 155

Tinea manuum Superficial fungal infection of the palms usually presents with erythema and whitish scale, predominantly in the palmar creases. It is almost always associated with tinea pedis. Generally tinea manuum involves one hand, but if both, is not symmetrical. The causative organism is usually *Trichophyton rubrum*. The condition may be treated with either topical imidazole creams or with oral griseofulvin. On the dorsa of the hands, the infecting fungi are more likely to be those that cause tinea corporis elsewhere.

Dermatophytids Fungal infections are sometimes accompanied by cutaneous eruptions that are the result of sensitization to the products of the fungi. Such cutaneous effects are called *dermatophytids* and are sterile of the fungi. Dermatophytids are papular and vesicular lesions, commonly on the hands. They usually stem from fungal infections of the foot that have become inflamed or irritated. The palmar blisters in this photograph are the result of such an event.

Figure 156

Figure 157

Tinea versicolor   This title designates a superficial fungal infection (*tinea*) that changes color (*versicolor*). The causative organism was originally called *Malassezia furfur* and is now called *Pityrosporum orbiculare*. Tinea versicolor typically causes numerous patchy scaling macules on the upper chest and back, proximal arms, and neck. Facial involvement may occur. The lesions may be hypopigmented, as illustrated here, or brown-orange in color, depending on the skin color of the patient and the degree of recent sun exposure. The organism is believed to prevent either the formation of melanin

or the transfer of melanosomes into keratinocytes. The formation of azelaic acid is another suggested mechanism for the resultant hypopigmentation. Although tinea versicolor usually makes its appearance after puberty, it can develop in childhood and is occasionally seen in breast-fed infants. Tinea versicolor is usually asymptomatic but may itch slightly. The organism cannot be cultured, but diagnosis is aided by the orange or brown glow of lesional skin under a Wood's light, and the "spaghetti and meatballs" appearance of clustered hyphae and spores on potassium hydroxide preparation.

Figure 158

Figure 159

Tinea versicolor   Illustrated here are small scaly macules, which are in this case darker than the surrounding skin. There are several approaches to the treatment of tinea versicolor. Small areas of involvement can be eradicated by use of an imidazole cream. In patients with more extensive disease, the best approach is the use of a selenium sulfide or sodium thiosulfate lotion. Patients should be forewarned that treatment of tinea versicolor does not diminish the very high rate of recurrence and that the return to normal skin color may be delayed weeks to months after the completion of therapy.

Tinea nigra   This is an infection of the stratum corneum, commonly on a palm, that is caused by the dematiaceous fungus *Exophalia (Cladosporium) werneckii*. It occurs most commonly in tropical regions. The clinical appearance is a tan-to-black discoloration with sharp borders which enlarge slowly. It can be mistaken for a melanocytic nevus, melanoma, or simple artifact. The correct diagnosis can be confirmed by KOH examination or fungal culture. Treatment consists of a keratolytic lotion or topical imidazole cream.

Figure 160

Tinea imbricata   Tinea imbricata is a superficial fungal in-fection of the glabrous skin that is seen in a number of tropical countries. The causative organism is *Trichophyton concentricum*. Brown papules evolve into annular plaques. As the infection continues, many concentric ring lesions develop, which resemble the patterning of a tortoise shell. Griseofulvin is an effective therapy but relapses occur.

Figure 161

Favus   This chronic form of tinea capitis is caused by *Trichophyton schoenleinii*. It occurs in parts of Europe, Africa, and South America, and also in some rural areas of the United States and Canada. Pictured here are the typical scaly patches seen in favus. The yellowish cup-like crusts, called *scutula,* are a distinctive part of this disease. The coalescent crusts form a plaque that emits a characteristic mousy order. This form of fungal infection of the scalp may persist into adult life.

Figure 162

Chromoblastomycosis   The particolored granulomatous process here illustrated is of 12 years' duration. It started as a small nodule, developed slowly into a verrucous mass, and acquired satellite extensions. The condition, so reminiscent of a tuberculous process, is a deep fungal infection caused by species of *Phialophora, Fonsecaea,* and *Cladosporium,* which are indigenous to South America and other geographic areas with warm climates. Lesions that are too large for surgical excision are treated with combinations of systemic flucytosine, amphotericin B, and ketoconazole.

Figure 163

Coccidioidomycosis   This disease, caused by the dimorphic fungus *Coccidioides immitis,* is endemic to the southwestern United States and parts of Central and South America. Most individuals in those areas develop the disease as an incon-sequential upper respiratory infection. However, severe dis-seminated disease can follow pulmonary infection and may involve the skin. In this case, the lesions are typically abscesses, nodules, or verrucous and inflammatory plaques. Primary infection of the skin, which is rare, is accompanied by regional lymphadenopathy. Amphotericin B is the custom-ary treatment.

Figure 164

Figure 165

Sporotrichosis Cutaneous infection with *Sporothrix schenckii* is a disease with worldwide distribution. The majority of cases are seen in Central and South America, but outbreaks in the United States occur. The disease affects both children and adults and occurs when the causative fungus, in either contaminated soil or plant materials, contacts traumatized skin. The thorn of a rose bush may provide both the organism and a site of entry, and there have been outbreaks among children playing among bales of hay. Pictured here is the most common form of sporotrichosis, the lymphocutaneous

type. It causes an ulcerated lesion at the site of inoculation (Fig. 164) and a string of nodules or ulcerations along the lines of lymphatic drainage (Fig. 165). These tender secondary lesions may become chronic and extend into subcutaneous tissues. Very rarely, and especially in the immunocompromised host, disseminated or systemic sporotrichosis follows cutaneous infection. Diagnosis of sporotrichosis can be confirmed by culture of exudate or tissue from the skin lesions on Sabouraud's agar.

Figure 166

Figure 167

Sporotrichosis This figure illustrates a somewhat less common form of the disease, fixed cutaneous sporotrichosis. The patient fell on rocks while playing in the country and sustained abrasions on an arm and elbow. *Sporothrix schenckii* was cultured from the crusted plaques in both locations. In this clinical form, the deep fungal infection remains confined to one area of the skin and has no tendency toward lymphatic spread. Treatment for all forms of cutaneous sporotrichosis consists of oral potassium iodide for a period of 4–6 weeks.

Histopathology of sporotrichosis Sporotrichosis is the most common deep fungal infection in which the skin is the portal of infection. The well-developed primary complex in the skin is clinically a chancriform or verrucous lesion that histologically shows epidermal hyperplasia and a dermal inflammatory infiltrate composed of neutrophils, mononuclear cells, and multinucleated giant cells, among which the infecting microorganism can sometimes be identified in the form of budding round bodies.

Figure 168

Figure 169

Candidiasis (moniliasis) Cutaneous infection with *Candida albicans* tends to occur in areas that are chronically moist, warm, and macerated. For this reason, candida is among the most common causes of diaper dermatitis. An early diaper rash in Fig. 168 illustrates some of the distinctive features of monilial infection. Note the confluent glistening beefy-red erythema which begins in the perianal skin and spreads by local extension. There are numerous small satellite lesions. If untreated, this rash will go on to involve the gluteal folds, buttocks and inner thighs. More extensive involvement is seen in Fig. 169; note the peripheral scaling and again the satellite lesions. On occasion, these peripheral pustules and papules will involve the entire abdomen and back. Diagnosis of cutaneous candidiasis can be confirmed by KOH preparation or by fungal culture. Treatment consists of the use any imidazole cream or nystatin. The several preparations that also contain a fluorinated topical steroid are not required for this condition and may lead to adverse local side effects.

Figure 170

Figure 171

Candidiasis (moniliasis) The angles of the mouth are also places where intertriginous conditions favor the overgrowth of ubiquitous *Candida albicans,* streptococci, staphylococci, and other ordinarily saprophytic but facultatively pathogenic microorganisms. The condition produced at the angles of the mouth (Fig. 170) is called *perlèche* or *angular stomatitis.* From such a beginning or even without it, the lips themselves may become involved in the manner pictured in Fig. 171. These conditions are not to be confused with vitamin deficiencies, which are often overdiagnosed. Perlèche is more likely to be a mixed infection with *C. albicans* and bacteria. Therefore, treatment should be with a preparation that contains both an antimonilial agent like nystatin and a topical antibiotic. Candidal cheilitis is more difficult to treat and requires persistent application of a candicidal agent. Candidiasis in children with immunologic deficiency is particularly difficult to treat.

Figure 172

Figure 173

Chronic mucocutaneous candidiasis The immunologic inability to handle *Candida albicans* infection results in recurrent and severe infection of the mucous membranes, skin, and nails. Affected children have T-cell deficiencies due to a wide variety of underlying causes but manifest their mucocutaneous disease in similar fashion. Illustrated here are chronic perlèche and candidal cheilitis (Fig. 172) and a circumscribed, erythematous, and hyperkeratotic candidal rash in the diaper area (Fig. 173). Both areas of involvement in these patients have been resistant to conventional anti-

monilial therapies. Chronic mucocutaneous candidiasis can also occur as an autosomal recessive syndrome, with no associated abnormalities. Early in their course, these children may be indistinguishable from those with profound immune deficiency disorders such as Swiss-type agammaglobulinemia, DiGeorge's syndrome, and Nezelof's syndrome. An identical clinical picture of unusual and persistent mucocutaneous monilial infection may be the presenting feature of infection with the human immunodeficiency virus.

Figure 174

Figure 175

Chronic mucocutaneous candidiasis Chronic mucocutaneous candidiasis may, in some patients, lead to granuloma formation in the areas of infection. The face is a common site for the formation of these indurated and hyperkeratotic plaques. Note how the lesions on the forehead of the patient in Fig. 174 resemble some forms of tuberculosis cutis, sporotrichosis, and chromoblastomycosis previously pictured and described. Figure 175 illustrates typical nail involvement in chronic mucocutaneous candidiasis. Patients develop swelling and tenderness of the proximal and lateral nail folds. Even-

tually, the nails become brittle and discolored and may be destroyed by the process. Treatment with oral ketoconazole is often effective. The use of intravenous amphotericin B and flucytosine should be reserved for nonresponsive cases. Some patients with acrodermatitis enteropathica (zinc deficiency) and certain children with iron deficiency develop chronic mucocutaneous candidiasis. Dietary or parenteral replacement of the deficient mineral, as required, leads to resolution of the candidal infections.

Figure 176

Figure 177

Chronic mucocutaneous candidiasis In many patients, chronic mucocutaneous candidiasis is part of an autoimmune syndrome which has profound effects on the endocrine system. Hypoparathyroidism is the most common of these autoimmune syndromes and is present in more than 80 percent of the children with chronic mucocutaneous candidiasis. The sparse brittle hair (Fig. 176) and the deforming effect of chronic hypocalcemia on tooth formation (Fig. 177) are both features of hypoparathyroidism. Other endocrine disorders that may be associated with chronic mucocutaneous candidiasis include hypoadrenocorticism, gonadal insufficiency, and thyroid abnormalities. Alopecia areata and vitiligo may also occur in these patients. Children with the so-called candidiasis endocrinopathy syndrome have the same nail, skin, and mucous membrane involvement as do children with chronic mucocutaneous candidiasis from other causes. The onset of these manifestations usually occurs in early childhood, and the endocrine disease develops during adolescence.

Figure 178

Figure 179

Congenital cutaneous candidiasis The presence of a generalized candidal dermatitis at birth is the result of intrauterine infection. Typically, erythematous papulovesicles and macules evolve into pustules and areas of superficial desquamation over a period of 6 to 8 days. The characteristic lesions frequently involve the palms and soles and may be accompanied by paronychiae and true nail involvement. In contrast to neonatal candidiasis (acquired during passage through an infected birth canal), the diaper area and oral mucosa tend to be spared. If congenital candidiasis involves only the skin, the disease follows a benign course. Infants with low birth weight or respiratory distress may develop disseminated infection and require systemic therapy.

7

Metazoal Diseases

Figure 180

Figure 181

Insect "bites" Many effects of metazoal parasitism are attributed to bites. Some metazoa (insects in a loose sense) do indeed bite and others sting, but what we frequently designate as insect bite is attachment for feeding. The result of such attachment looks like a bite and is sooner or later attended by pain, itching, or stinging. True bites and stings, however, are instantly painful; many have immediate or late, more baleful effects; and most are generally inflicted in self-defense or seemingly wanton offense, not for feeding. At-

tachment for feeding is parasitism that may be silent for a while and then variably symptomatic. In a given region, common, indigenous metazoa that cause cutaneous effects by a bite, sting, or attachment for feeding may be recognized or guessed from signs and symptoms. The two illustrations are representative: Fig. 180 may be guessed with reasonable correctness to be mosquito "bites" and Fig. 181, flea bites. We use quotation marks to suggest that the proboscis of a mosquito is not a true biting part. Fleas may nip.

Figure 182

Figure 183

Insect "bites" The mark of mosquito feeding is usually recognized easily because the season is right; the actual event is frequently seen as well as felt; often it is interrupted by a slap which, when successful, results in a dead assailant; and the clinical and symptomatic consequences are familiar. Figure 180 shows the type of pruritic, urticarial, or edematous lesion caused by mosquitoes. Figure 181 and Figs. 182 and 183 are characteristic of "bites" of insects that feed, browse, and feed again. Bedbugs and fleas are such insects. The

marks tend to be aligned in rows of two or three. In the case of the mosquito, the lesions may be one, few, or many depending on the insensitivity, foolhardiness, or defenselessness of the subject assailed. In the case of the bedbug, the number of lesions will depend on the number harbored and the immobility or restlessness and ineffable attractiveness of sleepers. Commonly only one of two or more contiguous bedfellows is afflicted.

Figure 184

Insect "bites" When a subject has been bitten, stung, or fed upon, the consequent lesion may be typical at the time and in course to resolution, or may be modified by scratching, secondary infection, or idiosyncratic host response. Lesions in Fig. 184 may well have been caused by mosquitoes, bedbugs, or fleas, but instead of the usual central punctum and surrounding erythema and edema, a summit of vesiculation has developed, probably signifying more-than-average host response as a result of previous sensitization.

Figure 185

Dermatitis caused by the common carpet beetle The common carpet beetle is not common in modern, well-sanitated homes, and even where it is abundant, effects from it are not common. Nevertheless, on occasion, the crawl of the insect on an unwary individual leaves its marks as wheals, papulovesicles, or bullae. The figure shows just such an event in the form of large, flaccid blisters. The three lesions in a line record the walk of a creature and the deposition of its irritant principle.

Figure 186

Insect "bites" Insect assaults on ordinarily well-covered parts of the body are special. The body louse lives in the seams of garments and comes onto the body to feed. The marks of its sojourns are scratches produced by the itchy victim. Certain insects creep under clothes and bite when they reach a point of restriction like a garter or belt. Figure 186 shows bite marks and vast edema on the penis. The assaulting insect may have been an ordinary one that merely took advantage of a child left undressed and unguarded.

Figure 187

Spider bites Spiders, timid creatures for all their fierce looks, would rather entertain insects in their parlors than attack man. The tarantula is more dangerous in fable than in fact. Two spiders can deliver painful bites and serious venenation if frightened or cornered: the black widow spider (*Latrodectus mactans*) and the brown recluse spider (*Loxosceles reclusa*). The bite of the latter is illustrated. It is a hemorrhagic bleb; in time it will become a necrotic ulcer. The patient will be severely sickened.

Figure 188

Tick bite Tick infestation occurs when the female soft or hard tick inserts her proboscis into the skin in order to withdraw blood. The site of attachment may develop into an erythematous nodule, and persistent pruritus may result if tick parts are left within the skin. Although most tick bites are insignificant, these insects may cause tick paralysis and are the vectors of Rocky Mountain spotted fever (Figs. 136, 137) and erythema chronicum migrans (Lyme disease) (Figs. 60 and 61).

Figure 189

Histopathology of insect bites and stings Clinical and histopathologic responses to bites and stings of insects vary from urticarial edema to long-enduring inflammation. The latter is the more important because it consists of cellular infiltration in the dermis and may suggest malignancy. In the photomicrograph, one sees epidermal thinning and crusting, hemorrhage in the upper cutis, and a heavy infiltrate of pleomorphic cells that simulates a lymphoma.

Figure 190

Scabies Infection of the skin by the human scabies mite (*Sarcoptes scabiei* var. *hominis*) is an extremely common skin disease of childhood. Numerous other species of mites that are obligatory parasites of dogs, cats, mice, and fowl or that subsist on food (cheese, grain, and other cereals) may also infest humans. Figure 190 shows a mild infestation with a mite ordinarily obligatory to dogs; Fig. 191 shows infestation with the human itch mite. The infant with scabies illustrated

Figure 191

here has numerous excoriated papules and a diffuse eczematous dermatitis. In infants, scabies frequently involves the entire cutaneous surface, including the face. Inflammatory nodular lesions involving the axillae and the diaper area are particularly typical of scabies in the very young child. These lesions may coexist with burrows, papules, vesicles, pustules, and areas of crusting.

Figure 192

Figure 193

Scabies The location of primary lesions is often helpful in establishing the diagnosis of scabies. In older children and adolescents, the most common sites for the intensely pruritic lesions are the anterior axillary lines, the inner aspect of the upper arm, the areolae, the penis, the wrists and interdigital webs, and the ankles. In young children, the palms (Fig. 192) and soles are additional sites of predilection. Figure 193 is an illustration of the infestation in the anterior axillary lines.

The undisturbed lesion of scabies is a red papule that is a shallow burrow directly beneath the stratum corneum. It contains the gravid female and her young. When scabies is widespread and in typical areas of distribution, diagnosis can be made with surety on clinical grounds alone. In sporadic cases and when lesions are few, the top of a primary lesion may be gently shaved or scraped off into a drop of mineral oil and examined microscopically for the presence of mites.

Figure 194

Figure 195

Scabies Figure 194 shows typical lesions of scabies on the lower part of the abdomen, the penis, and the dorsum of the hand. The preferred treatment of scabies is a single application of lindane lotion, from the neck down and under the fingernails. The use of this medication in infants, however, remains somewhat controversial. An effective alternative in this age group is the twice daily application of 6% sulfur ointment for 3 days. The application of any scabicide must be accompanied by the thorough laundering of all recently worn clothing and of bed linen, which may still contain mites or eggs. Figure

195 is a photograph of so-called Norwegian scabies. Individuals with this form of the disease develop thick areas of heavy crusting. Favored locations for the hyperkeratotic plaques include the elbows, knees, scalp, and buttocks. The areas of involvement contain numerous mites, and therefore the disease is highly contagious. Norwegian scabies occurs most commonly in patients with Down's syndrome and among those who are debilitated or who suffer from an immune deficiency.

Figure 196

Figure 197

Pediculosis capitis   The head louse is a six-legged wingless insect that is the smallest of the three human lice. It is adapted to live in the hair of the scalp only and lives by feeding on blood. The female louse lays approximately 4 eggs per day and has a life span of 2 to 4 weeks. She uses a gluey substance to attach the egg cases or nits to the hair. The diagnosis of pediculosis capitis is suggested by the presence of itching in the posterior scalp or signs of redness or folliculitis at the nape of the neck. Diagnosis is confirmed by the presence of nits, which, even when sparse, are easily recognized with hand-lens magnification. The reader is advised to use a hand lens on Fig. 196, which will reveal the nits well. The nit can also be recognized by examining an infested hair under the microscope (Fig. 197). Treatment is simple and consists of either 1% lindane shampoo or a permethrin cream rinse. Remaining nits may be removed with a fine-tooth comb, aided by the application of an equal mixture of vinegar and water.

Figure 198

Figure 199

Pediculosis corporis   The body louse belongs to the genus *Pediculus*; it is larger and broader than the head louse. Whereas the head louse infests the skin of the scalp, the body louse does not live on the body. It lives in the seams of undergarments and comes onto the body only to feed. Clinically, one sees marks of feeding and excoriations; the lice themselves can be found in the clothes. Treatment consists of disinfestation of clothing and bedding and the application of a pediculicide to the patient.

Pediculosis pubis   The pubic louse (*Phthirus pubis*) is aptly called the crab louse. Examined under the microscope, this insect is broad like a crab and has legs that look like claws. On the skin, the louse looks like a brown fleck and may be mistaken for a freckle. Nits are also easily seen grossly, and better by hand-lens magnification. The illustration is a good representation. Infestation may also occur in the eyelashes and axillary hair. Treatment consists of lindane shampoo or a variety of over-the-counter products which contain a pyrethrin.

Figure 200

Figure 201

Myiasis   The term for infestation with the larvae of flies is pronounced mī′yĕ-sīs or mī-ī′ ĕ-sīs. In this condition flies deposit fertilized ova upon neglected wounds or under onycholytic nails. The infestation is usually a sign of poor hygiene. *Dermatobia hominis, Wohlfahrtia vigil,* and several other species of botflies and warble flies may foster their young in

this way. Figure 200 shows a cutaneous lesion but does not reveal the larvae, which can be better seen in movement in vivo by the naked eye. Figure 201 shows a larva clearly. In most cases, the larvae can be easily removed mechanically under local anesthesia. Antibiotics may be needed to treat secondary infection.

Figure 202

Figure 203

Caterpillar dermatitis   The hairs of caterpillars and moths may produce pruritic or painful inflammatory skin lesions. The puss caterpillar and brown-tail moth are the most common offenders. The toxin on the spines and hairs of these insects causes an irritant dermatitis. The resultant lesions, which are sometimes seen in linear array, may be papular or urticarial, and are accompanied by itching or stinging. Systemic symptoms are rare but may occur. The hairs may be seen microscopically in skin scrapings. Treatment is purely symptomatic.

Dermatitis caused by blister beetles   There are several species of beetles (order Coleoptera) that secrete onto their bodies cantharidin or some other vesicant substance. The crawl of the so-called blister beetles smears their irritant substances on the skin, causing the edema and blistering illustrated in the figure. Treatment with cool compresses and topical antibiotics to prevent superinfection is usually adequate.

Figure 204

Figure 205

Cutaneous schistosomiasis (swimmer's or seabather's itch)
Collections of swampy water or of shallow water along lake
or river shorelines may be infested with schistosomes. A
dermatitis results when these flukes or cercariae adhere to
the skin by their ventral suckers and penetrate. Pruritus
begins within a few minutes of exposure and is accompanied
by an urticarial reaction at the site of entry. Subsequently,
numerous erythematous papules and pustules evolve, each
at the location of a schistosome. These intensely itchy lesions

tend to resolve spontaneously over a period of 1–2 weeks.
The severity of the dermatitis may increase in subsequent
episodes. The pictures show the cutaneous process well.
Figure 204 shows lesions under the bathing trunks, and Fig.
205 shows them in sharper detail on the thigh. Like any
intensely pruritic condition, excoriations and secondary infection are complications. Treatment consists of antipruritics,
and antibiotics when superinfection occurs.

Figure 206

Figure 207

The sting of the Portuguese man-of-war   One of the most
painful effects on skin is the consequence of attack by oceanic
hydrozoans known as Portuguese men-of-war, which are
amazing for their size, brilliant color, and power to induce
whealing. They have a small float which buoys them up and
from which hang tentacles of great size. The wrap of these
tentacles results in linear stripes, which look like whip lashes,
caused not by the force of their swing but from deposition
of urticariogenic and irritant substances.

The effect of contact with a sea urchin   Sea urchins are a
gastronomic delight when prepared properly, but a cutaneous
torture when stepped on unprepared. The echinoids have
spines that in some species are several inches long. Driven
into skin when one steps or falls on or brushes against the
creatures, the hard spines break and lodge in skin. Pain is
inevitable, and secondary infection is nearly inevitable if they
are left. Nothing but tedious and meticulous extraction of
every one of dozens, possibly scores, is required for relief.

Figure 208

Figure 209

Larva migrans (creeping eruption) Infestation of the skin with larvae of certain helminths, notably *Ancylostoma braziliense,* is common on the southern coast of the United States as well as in some other parts of the world. Helminths like *A. braziliense* infest the intestines of animals, particularly the dog, whose excreta contain larvae that have remarkable capacity to enter unbroken skin. Attaining the interior just below the stratum corneum, the immature forms move in a serpentine, erratic way, creating long channels. The larvae are sometimes barely discernible at the ends of the channels in the direction of travel. The feet, buttocks, arms, hands, and back are common sites of lodgment and lesions. The pictures show characteristic linear lesions on a foot (Fig. 208) and on buttocks and labia in an infant (Fig. 209) who was unwittingly placed on a contaminated beach or lawn. Treatment consists of the topical application of thiabendazole.

Figure 210

Figure 211

Onchocerciasis *Onchocerca volvulus,* like *Tunga penetrans, Dracunculus medinensis, Wuchereria bancroftii,* and *Loa loa,* is limited to parts of the developing world. All these metazoa infest deeply and are difficult to eradicate. The filarial elephantiasis caused by *Wuchereria bancroftii,* the edema (Calabar swellings) about the eyes caused by the "African eye worm" (*Loa loa*), and the interdigital nodule, usually between toes, that harbors yards of the guinea worm (*Dracunculus medinensis*) are endemic to varying regions of Africa, South America, and Asia. Onchocerciasis is seen commonly in parts of Mexico. The metazoan that causes this disease is often found in the scalp and around the eyes, where infection may have serious consequences. Figure 211 is a lumpy lesion on the scalp, caused by the adult worm. Figure 210 shows less discernible lesions on the chest. These are caused by the organism in its microfilarial phase. The oral medication Ivermectin (Merck) is the drug of choice.

Allergic, Eczematous, Irritant, and Light-Related Dermatoses

Figure 212

Figure 213

Papular urticaria   This is a pruritic dermatosis that is causally related to bites by mosquitoes, fleas, or other insects. Children with this common disorder tend to have recurrent episodes during the spring and summer months. The lesions consist of firm erythematous papules, sometimes with surrounding wheals. They favor exposed areas, especially the anterior lower extremities and lower arms. The individual papules are often excoriated and are sometimes impetiginized. The lesions tend to last for several days to weeks but will persist longer if chronically scratched or rubbed. Papular urticaria is more common among children with the atopic diathesis and represents a hypersensitivity reaction to the assaulting arthropod. Treatment consists of shake lotions, topical steroids, and antihistamines. The elimination of the offending insect from the household environment is helpful but will not prevent encounters during outdoor play.

Figure 214

Figure 215

Prurigo mitis   This dermatosis occurs exclusively in children with the atopic diathesis, i.e., either a personal or family history of atopic disease. The disease consists of chronic, pruritic papules which tend to favor the abdomen, extensor extremities, and buttocks. The lesions become excoriated, impetiginized and lichenified over time. The relation between papular urticaria and prurigo mitis is somewhat unclear. Some observers believe that this condition begins with papular urticaria and is a chronic form of that disorder. In any case, children with prurigo mitis seem to have a more chronic and persistent dermatosis than those with simple papular urticaria.

Figure 216

Figure 217

Atopic dermatitis   This condition is the most common of all pediatric dermatoses. For the majority of patients, onset occurs during infancy. The classic clinical appearance in this age group is illustrated in Fig. 216. There are symmetrical patches of erythema, exudation, and scale involving the cheeks and chin. It is not unusual to also see widespread involvement of the trunk and extensor extremities during infancy; the diaper area is most often spared. Figure 217 shows similar distribution in an older child. In this case,

impetiginization may be contributing to the crusted appearance of the lesions. Pruritus is a cardinal feature of atopic dermatitis and may be evidenced in the infant by irritability, scratching, and rubbing against nearby objects. Atopic dermatitis is an inherited disorder. Children with the disease most often have a family history of the atopic diathesis (either atopic dermatitis, asthma, or allergic rhinitis) and may themselves manifest asthma or allergic respiratory disease.

Figure 218

Figure 219

Atopic dermatitis   When the diagnosis of atopic dermatitis is in doubt, the search for associated clinical findings is often helpful. Two such near pathognomonic cutaneous signs of atopic dermatitis are pictured here. The Dennie-Morgan line (Fig. 218) is a double fold under the eye which is seen in many children with atopic dermatitis. Figure 219 shows another telltale sign: a fissure at the junction of the pinna of

the ear and the face. Other associated findings related to atopic dermatitis include pityriasis alba (Figs. 228 and 229), keratosis pilaris (Figs. 252–254), lichen spinulosus (Figs. 312 and 313), and ichthyosis vulgaris (Figs. 394–396). Children with atopic dermatitis are also frequently noted to have hyperlinear palms and soles. Keratoconjunctivitis and cataracts may occur in the child with atopic dermatitis.

Figure 220

Figure 221

Atopic dermatitis (cont.)   During childhood, the most common locations of atopic dermatitis are the antecubital and popliteal fossae and the posterior neck. Pictured here are children in whom involvement is more widespread. The lesions show the characteristic erythema, oozing, and crusting of acute atopic dermatitis. This appearance correlates with the histopathology. Spongiosis and intracellular edema are cardinal features of acute lesions; chronic plaques show acanthosis and hyperkeratosis. The pathogenesis of atopic

dermatitis remains a mystery. Patients with the disease seem to have altered autonomic function and increased plasma histamine levels. Many have elevated levels of IgE, but some are completely normal in this respect. Finally, there is evidence of diminished cell-mediated immunity and poly-morphonuclear chemotaxis in atopics. However, none of these observations has as yet provided a basis for understanding the chronic and recurrent skin lesions of atopic dermatitis.

Figure 222

Figure 223

Atopic dermatitis   These are illustrations of atopic dermatitis on the elbow (Fig. 222) and in a popliteal space (Fig. 223) in a 5-year-old child. As mentioned above, the latter is a very common site for involvement in this age group. The majority of children with atopic dermatitis experience resolution of their disease and have normal skin as adults. However, the severe pruritus and the unpleasant appearance of the skin which accompany the exacerbations of this condition can be extremely troubling to parent and child alike. The role of diet

in the treatment of atopic dermatitis remains controversial. Despite evidence that some atopic children display a significant histamine response to some foods, it is fair to say that the majority of children with the disease do not respond to modifications of their diet. However, any foods that cause an obvious worsening of the condition should be avoided. Occasionally, food allergy in the atopic child may even be manifested by the rapid evolution of contact urticaria on the face and hands.

Figure 224

Figure 225

Atopic dermatitis Figure 224 illustrates an area that is scaly and lichenified. Figure 225 shows atopic dermatitis involving one toe. The treatment of atopic dermatitis should include the establishment of a routine of skin care that maintains adequate hydration of the skin. Frequent bathing and the use of alkali soaps is to be avoided. Parents should be encouraged to apply a lubricating ointment to the child's skin several times a day. Topical corticosteroid ointments are currently the mainstay of medical management. Many children do well with proper use of the milder, non-fluorinated ointments, but some require stronger preparations for brief periods of time. The dangers of local atrophy and stria formation and of systemic absorption must be considered carefully with the use of the stronger formulations. The fluorinated corticosteroids should never be used on the face or in intertriginous areas. Important adjuncts to therapy include antihistamines, and, occasionally, a brief course of oral antibiotics to reduce skin colonization with streptococcus and staphylococcus.

Figure 226

Figure 227

Juvenile plantar dermatitis Figure 226 shows erythema and fissuring on the weight-bearing surface of the foot. This disorder, which tends to be worse in the winter months, is called *juvenile plantar dermatitis*. It is much more common in children with atopic dermatitis. Juvenile plantar dermatitis, which has also been called *wet-dry foot syndrome,* is caused by excessive sweating of the feet in occlusive footwear and rapid drying in a low humidity environment. The use of emollient ointments is extremely helpful.

Summer prurigo Illustrated here are fine, erythematous, and flesh-colored papules on the elbows. This pruritic eruption, termed *summer prurigo* or *summertime pityriasis,* occurs most commonly but not exclusively in children with the atopic diathesis. The rash is seen most frequently between the ages of 4 and 10 and tends to recur seasonally in the late spring or early summer. Some children also have lesions on the knees and dorsa of the hands.

Figure 228

Figure 229

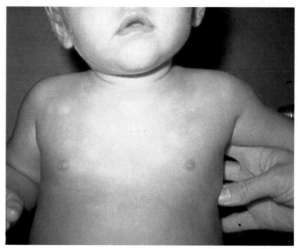

Pityriasis alba   This is a condition which is characterized by blotchy areas of hypopigmentation, with or without scale. The lesions are usually asymptomatic. In older children, the cheeks are a favored location, but in infants the process may be more generalized. Both figures illustrate how the borders of the lesions tend to fade into the surrounding normal skin. This contrasts with vitiligo (Figs. 724–727), another common cause of pigment loss. In vitiligo, the areas of involvement

tend to be a whiter white and are more sharply demarcated. Pityriasis alba is more common among children with atopic dermatitis and probably represents a form of postinflammatory hypopigmentation. There may or may not be a preceding inflammatory dermatosis in the same area. It is important to reassure parent and child that the loss of pigment is temporary and that complete restoration of normal skin color will occur. The use of a mild topical steroid may speed the process.

Figure 230

Figure 231

Pompholyx (dishydrotic eczema)   This is a chronic recurrent eruption of the hands and feet that is often accompanied by severe pruritus. It is considerably more common among individuals with an atopic history or with a family history of atopic disease. Figures 230 and 231 show a number of deep-seated vesicles and pustules on the palm and thumb. Small, firm vesicles along the sides of the fingers are a particularly

common clinical sign. At times, bullae may occur. Patients who develop pompholyx often tend to have hyperhidrosis of the hands and feet. Some observers note that episodes of the disease are brought on by stress. Management of this condition is best achieved by the use of drying agents and topical corticosteroid creams or ointments with or without tar.

Figure 232

Figure 233

Palmoplantar pustulosis This chronic condition is characterized by erythematous plaques which are studded with multiple small pustules. The lesions are confined to the palms and soles, and onset may occur during childhood. The etiology of palmoplantar pustulosis is a mystery, and early theories that tried to correlate this disease with chronic occult infection (so-called pustular bacterid) have largely been discarded. Although pustular eruptions of the palms and soles are seen in many patients with psoriasis, the patients with palmoplantar

pustulosis do not go on to develop psoriasis in other areas. Adolescents with palmoplantar pustulosis sometimes develop recurrent multifocal osteomyelitis. This is a chronic condition in which episodes of bone pain are found to be caused by localized areas of biopsy-proven osteomyelitis, usually in the long bones or sternum. Characteristically, repeated cultures of the bone marrow are negative. The osteomyelitis and pustular dermatosis tend to flare spontaneously, but the relationship between the two conditions is not known.

Figure 234

Figure 235

Lichen striatus This is a common and benign, self-limited childhood dermatosis which is easily diagnosed by its classic appearance. Onset is usually between the ages of 3 and 10, and it is rare in young infants, adolescents, and adults. The lesions consist of pink, flesh-colored or slightly hypopigmented flat-topped papules which evolve in a linear array. As pictured in Fig. 234, the linear course of the papules may

eventually traverse the major part of an extremity. The area of involvement is often noted to become wider as it advances and may even include the nails. The lesions of lichen striatus are usually asymptomatic but may last 6 months to 1 year or even longer. The etiology of the condition is unknown. Treatment is not strictly necessary, but mild topical steroids tend to speed the process of resolution.

Figure 236

Figure 237

Allergic contact dermatitis This condition is a T-cell mediated delayed hypersensitivity response to a variety of different antigens. Acute lesions are characterized by erythema, vesiculation, and oozing, while chronic areas of involvement may be dry and lichenified. The diagnosis of allergic contact dermatitis is made simple when there is a clear history of exposure to an allergen or when the distribution of the lesions provides a strong clue. At other times, the identification of the causative agent can be very difficult. A number of different plants are capable of causing contact

dermatitis. By far the most common are members of the genus *Toxicodendron*: poison ivy, oak, and sumac. These are illustrations of contact dermatitis from poison ivy, the most common single cause of contact dermatitis in childhood. The linear array of vesicles and bullae in Fig. 236 reflects the pattern in which the resin was transferred from leaf to skin. Figure 237 shows a more diffuse reaction. Children who experience recurrent episodes of this phytodermatitis should be encouraged to learn to recognize the causative plants.

Figure 238

Figure 239

Allergic contact dermatitis These photographs illustrate two other common causes of allergic contact dermatitis. The young girl in Fig. 238 has developed an area of vesiculation and crusting because she is allergic to the nickel in her earrings. The same rash may develop under the metal buttons on blue jeans or beneath a wristwatch. Coating the surface of these metallic objects with clear nail polish will sometimes protect the skin from the allergen. In Fig. 239, a band of erythema and vesiculation has appeared on a thigh of a girl who has become sensitized to some component of rubber in

an undergarment. Synthetic rubber contains many potential allergens, but the most common offenders are antioxidants and rubber accelerators. The treatment of allergic contact dermatitis is based on the successful identification and avoidance of the skin allergen. When the cause is not obvious, the use of a standard patch test kit may be of enormous benefit. The resolution of acute episodes of contact dermatitis is hastened by the application of topical corticosteroids; a brief course of oral prednisone is sometimes indicated in widespread disease.

Figure 240

Allergic contact dermatitis The allergic contact dermatitis in this figure was caused by a sandal. Note how the eruption conforms, like a patch test, to the design of the thongs. Shoe dermatitis should be considered in any eczematous eruption on the dorsum of the foot in a child. The agent responsible for the rash in this photograph was a tanning agent or dye. The other common causes of shoe dermatitis are rubber and rubber accelerators, adhesives, and leather. If the allergen is correctly identified by patch testing, it is possible to select footwear that is tolerable.

Figure 241

Allergic contact dermatitis The picture is of a patch test with resorcinol, positive in the form of a vesicular reaction at 48 hours in a person who had become sensitive to it. Resorcinol is a common substance used in dermatologic preparations and in proprietary formulations sold over the counter. The same sort of reaction would occur in a person sensitive to mercury, benzocaine, formaldehyde, paraphenylenediamine, and many other substances used in formal prescriptions and proprietaries.

Figure 242

Figure 243

Allergic contact dermatitis Figure 242 illustrates the result of sensitization to an ingredient in lipstick. Lipstick cheilitis may be caused by indelible dyes, perfumes, or lanolin derivatives. The child in Fig. 243 has an allergic contact dermatitis resulting from the repeated application of a preparation containing neomycin. The development or worsening of an eczematous eruption after the use of a topical medication, either prescribed or over-the-counter, should alert the physician to the possibility of a contact dermatitis (dermatitis medicamentosa). In addition to neomycin, common offenders are the stabilizer ethylenediamine and the paraben preservatives.

Figure 244

Figure 245

Cutaneous effects of primary irritation   Irritant contact dermatitis is an eczematous eruption that results from the application of an irritating substance to the skin. Examples would include strong acids or alkalis, harsh soaps, and bleaches. In these cases, T-cell mediated allergy is not involved. The irritant in Fig. 244 is saliva. The child pictured here has developed a habit of licking his lips. Some children do this as compulsively as others suck their thumbs or bite their nails. Notice how the design of the inflammatory lesions conforms to the extent to which the lips can be drawn into the mouth or licked by the tongue. In Fig. 245, postinflammatory hyperpigmentation is shown in a child who has recovered from inflammation induced by chewing and blowing bubble gum.

Figure 246

Figure 247

Perioral dermatitis   This condition is a chronic eruption of fine papules and pustules located on the skin around the mouth and sometimes around the eyes and nose. The etiology of this condition is not completely understood, but in many children the use of topical corticosteroids seems either to cause or perpetuate the condition. In most instances, perioral dermatitis responds to oral tetracycline or erythromycin or to the topical application of ketoconazole or econazole. Topical steroids should be tapered and stopped. Rarely, as illustrated in Fig. 247, the lesions of perioral dermatitis may have a granulomatous appearance and histology and can be confused with sarcoid.

Figure 248

Intertrigo   Where skin is in natural apposition (for example, in the axillae, intergluteal folds, and neck folds) or where the skin is occluded, it is susceptible to the effects of wetness, higher temperature, friction, and accumulated debris. An area of slight erythema in the neck fold is illustrated here. The skin is superficially inflamed from excessive maceration of the stratum corneum, caused by retention of wetness from washing and insufficient drying or from retained sweat.

Figure 249

Irritant diaper dermatitis   The most common form of diaper dermatitis is related to the combination of moisture and friction. The result is illustrated in Fig. 249. Note the areas of involvement are folds of skin that are in direct apposition to the diaper itself; the skin creases tend to be spared. The bright erythema and shiny appearance of the involved skin are typical. Rashes of this type must be differentiated from candidiasis, seborrheic dermatitis, and psoriasis.

Figure 250

Erosive diaper dermatitis (dermatitis of Jacquet)   Inflammation that results from the precipitating factors of wetness, heat, friction, and debris in intertriginous places varies directly with the intensity and duration of those precipitating factors. The inflammation may be merely a slight erythema, a tumid, beefy redness with serous exudation, or an area of ulceration. The punched out ulcer illustrated here is typical of the erosive diaper dermatitis of Jacquet. This severe irritant dermatitis responds to the use of barrier creams and mild topical steroids.

Figure 251

Granuloma gluteale infantum   This term refers to a granulomatous eruption of infancy that is usually confined to the diaper area but may also involve other intertriginous parts. The lesions are typically large nodules with a red or purplish hue; their alarming appearance may falsely suggest the presence of a neoplasm. The cause of this dermatosis seems to be a combination of local inflammation and, sometimes, cutaneous candidiasis. It may be aggravated by the use of fluorinated topical steroids.

Figure 252

Figure 253

Keratosis pilaris This is an asymptomatic condition that is often familial and is sometimes associated with atopic dermatitis or ichthyosis vulgaris. Pictured here are typical lesions in the two most common areas of involvement, the lateral aspect of the upper arms and the anterior thighs. The lesions are fine keratotic papules; each represents a plug in the upper part of a hair follicle. The appearance of the involved areas is often likened to chicken skin or gooseflesh; the sensation on palpation is a grater-like roughness. Keratosis pilaris tends to worsen during the winter months and improves somewhat after puberty. Keratolytics and emollients are somewhat helpful.

Figure 254

Figure 255

Keratosis pilaris Children with keratosis pilaris sometimes develop the condition's typical follicular papules on the cheeks. When this occurs, there may also be erythema associated with the roughness. This condition is sometimes termed *keratosis pilaris rubra faciei*. Again, mild keratolytics are sometimes helpful.

Xerosis The accentuation of skin markings and fine scale illustrated here are typical of xerosis. The tendency toward dry skin tends to be inherited and is more common in families with a history of atopy. Low humidity, usually related to dry heat during the winter months, is an aggravating factor. Treatment of xerosis is aimed at rehydrating the stratum corneum. Emollients containing urea or lactic acid are particularly effective. Excessive bathing and the use of alkaline soaps must be avoided.

Figure 256

Figure 257

Polymorphous light eruption Patients with this condition develop papules, papulovesicles, or erythematous plaques in response to sun exposure. The lesions erupt anywhere from a few hours to several days after the subject is exposed to sunlight and seem to be a response to the UVB (290–320 nm) part of the action spectrum. Lesions are most often located on the face, upper chest, and exposed parts of the extremities. Ocular inflammation and cheilitis may also occur. Among North American and Latin American Indians, polymorphous light eruption tends to be a familial disease with childhood onset. Figure 256 shows an area of erythema and edema. The butterfly rash illustrated in Fig. 257 gives a sense that polymorphous light eruption can sometimes be difficult to differentiate from the cutaneous findings in systemic lupus erythematosus. Both immunofluorescence and serology are useful techniques in differentiating the two diseases. Sunscreens, antimalarial medications, topical corticosteroids, and psoralen with ultraviolet light (PUVA) are among the treatments used for polymorphous light eruption.

Figure 258

Figure 259

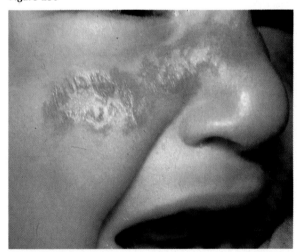

Photoallergic and phototoxic dermatitides In addition to sunburn and polymorphous light eruption, there are several other abnormal cutaneous reactions in which sunlight is part of the causative mechanism. Among these are photoallergic (Fig. 258) and phototoxic (Fig. 259) dermatitides. In the former, sensitization and subsequent clinical reactions develop to a topically applied or internally administered substance that has been activated to allergenicity by sunlight. The topical halogenated salicylanilides are among the most common causative agents in photoallergy. In phototoxic reactivity, no immunologic mechanism is involved, and the patient reacts as anyone would to a primary irritant. Phototoxic drugs and chemicals include some dyes, coal tar derivatives, and the psoralens. Drugs that may cause a phototoxic reaction include the sulfonamides, tetracyclines, and thiazides.

Berloque dermatitis (phytophotocontact dermatitis) This condition is a special kind of photoreaction in which the skin becomes slightly inflamed and quickly develops hyperpigmentation. The cutaneous changes are the result of contact with a photosensitizing chemical, followed immediately by sunlight. The most common causative agents are furocoumarins (psoralens). These figures illustrate the form of this condition which results from the application of a psoralen-

containing perfume, such as oil of bergamot. Note that the hyperpigmentation follows the exact distribution in which the perfume was applied. In addition to perfumes, a number of plants, grasses, fruits, and vegetables contain psoralen as a photosensitizer. The child who helps mother or father slice limes before a trip to the park may develop an identical eruption on the hands. Celery and parsley may present similar problems.

Figure 262

Figure 263

Actinic prurigo This title refers to a disease with onset in early childhood. Patients develop an intensely pruritic eruption in response to sunlight. The papules, vesicles, and crusted plaques tend to favor areas of exposed skin but may become generalized. The disease process is most severe during the late spring and summer. Illustrated in both figures is the inflammatory, pruritic dermatitis on a common location, the pinnae of the ears. The relationship between the disease

called *actinic prurigo* (or Hutchinson's summer prurigo) and polymorphous light eruption (Figs. 256, 257) has been an area of controversy. Some observers believe that the diseases are identical, but others feel that actinic prurigo is a distinct entity. Treatment for children with this clinical syndrome consists of maximal protection from sunlight. Topical steroids are of some benefit during exacerbations.

Papulosquamous, Lichenoid, and Perforating Disorders

Figure 264

Figure 265

Seborrheic dermatitis This title refers to a scaly, crusting, and erythematous eruption that favors areas where there are numerous sebaceous glands. It is most common in infancy (ages 2 to 12 weeks), when it tends to favor the scalp, diaper area, and intertriginal folds. Figure 264 is an illustration of the process in the scalp, where it is often referred to as *cradle cap*. Figure 265 shows seborrheic dermatitis in the diaper area. The photographs cannot convey the greasiness of the condition, and indeed at certain stages dry scaling rather than oiliness is predominant. A subset of infants with seborrheic

dermatitis will go on to develop atopic dermatitis, and, at times, it may be difficult to differentiate between these two conditions. Some basic principles are that the lesions of seborrheic dermatitis are usually well circumscribed, do not itch, and localize toward the scalp and intertriginal areas. The greasy red-orange scaliness of seborrheic dermatitis is somewhat helpful in differentiating this disorder from atopic dermatitis. Finally, seborrheic dermatitis has its onset early in infancy and usually resolves by 1 year of age; atopic dermatitis tends to begin later and to be more persistent.

Figure 266

Figure 267

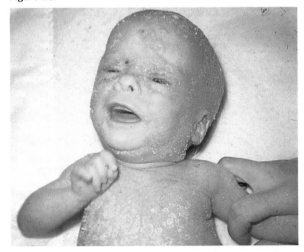

Seborrheic dermatitis Figure 266 shows seborrheic dermatitis in and around the axilla. Note the circumscribed salmon-colored lesions and the greasy character of the scale. Figure 267 shows a more extensive process that is nearly generalized and drier in scaly appearance. The cause of this very common condition remains unknown. Although it favors areas with an increased number of sebaceous glands, there is no evidence

that seborrheic dermatitis is a disease of sebaceous glands or is related to excessive sebum production. Some studies have suggested that the lipid composition of sebum in seborrheic dermatitis may be abnormal. Bacteria and yeasts are often present in areas of involvement, but neither *Candida albicans* nor *Pityrosporum ovale* has been shown to be an etiologic agent.

Figure 268

Figure 269

Seborrheic dermatitis Seborrheic dermatitis, common during infancy, is relatively unusual during later childhood. It resurfaces as a problem during adolescence and then seems to become progressively more common through adult life. The generalized seborrheic dermatitis of infancy gives way to a process that primarily involves the scalp, forehead, tarsal margins of the eyelids (blepharitis), ears, and nasolabial folds. Itching or vague discomfort sometimes accompanies the low-grade inflammation. Flares of the disease tend to occur during

the spring and fall seasons. Pictured in Fig. 268 are erythema and greasy scaling of the forehead and eyebrows. Figure 269 illustrates typical involvement of the nasolabial folds. Seborrheic dermatitis is easily controlled but not everlastingly curable. Treatment may consist of a sulfur and salicylic acid ointment or a mild topical steroid cream. The frequent use of tar shampoos is particulary helpful in the control of seborrheic dermatitis of the scalp.

Figures 270

Figure 271

Seborrheic dermatitis After puberty and in adulthood, seborrheic dermatitis occurs not only on the scalp and face but also on the chest, on the back, and in intertriginous spaces like the axillae, inframammary areas, groin, and intergluteal fold. Lesions on the chest and back are described as petaloid, i.e., flat and demarcated like petals; in intertriginous spaces, glistening redness is the appearance. The photograph shows the latter in an axilla.

Tinea amiantacea This title requires etymologic explanation. The *tinea* does not mean superficial fungal infection but rather a condition that resembles a superficial mycosis. *Amiantacea* means asbestos-like. The combination describes a superficial, scaly process that recalls the crumbling exfoliation of asbestos. Such an appearance occurs in the scalp in some cases of seborrheic dermatitis, psoriasis, tinea capitis, and pityriasis sicca (dandruff). The title is discarded as soon as a better diagnosis is made.

Figure 272

Figure 273

Psoriasis More than one-quarter of all individuals with psoriasis develop their disease during childhood or adolescence. The degree of involvement is extremely variable; some children develop only a few localized plaques while others suffer from generalized skin disease and severe arthritis. Pictured in Fig. 272 are the typical lesions of psoriasis; the plaques have a red-to-orange hue, are scaly, and are sharply demarcated from the surrounding skin. The symmetrical involvement of the knees is a common pattern; elbows and

buttocks are other favored locations for plaques like these. The distinctive character of the scale is best appreciated in Fig. 273. The scale is usually described as silvery or micaceous (resembling the mineral mica). When the scale is removed, pinpoint areas of bleeding (Auspitz sign) are uncovered. Each lesion of psoriasis represents an area of rapid epidermal cell turnover. The thickening of the involved epidermis and the overlying parakeratosis translate into the raised and scaly appearance of the involved skin.

Figure 274

Figure 275

Psoriasis In Fig. 274 we see typical areas of involvement on the glabrous skin of the neck and plaques of dense adherent scale in the scalp. Circumscribed areas of micaceous scale in the scalp are a common presenting sign of psoriasis. Figure 275 shows the scaling and thickening of the palms and soles that are very common in both children and adults with psoriasis. Therapy of psoriasis is based on the skillful use, either alone or in combination, of a number of therapeutic agents. The most effective are topical steroids, tars, keratolytics, and ultraviolet light. Children with simple plaque

psoriasis can often be managed with short contact anthralin preparations. When topical steroids are used, it is important to employ the least potent preparation as is effective and to avoid the use of fluorinated steroids on the face and in intertriginous areas. Preparations containing salicylic acid, a keratolytic, are especially useful for treatment of scalp psoriasis. Finally, careful exposure to sunlight during the summer months and artificial ultraviolet light at other times is enormously beneficial in selected patients with extensive involvement.

Figure 276

Figure 277

Psoriasis Pictured here are two more representations of common forms of psoriasis. In Fig. 276 the lesions consist of numerous papules, each covered with the typical silvery scales of psoriasis. This form of the condition, termed *guttate psoriasis,* is more common in childhood and may have an explosive onset. There is often a history of an antecedent upper respiratory infection, and streptococcal disease is of particular importance in triggering this eruption. The use of

oral antibiotics that are effective against streptococcus sometimes hastens the resolution of guttate psoriasis. Figure 277 illustrates psoriasis in the diaper area. When onset of the disease occurs during infancy, this is a very common area of involvement. It is postulated that the repeated irritation in this area constitutes a type of Koebner phenomenon. Scales are less in evidence because of the maceration that is inevitable in this location.

Figure 278

Figure 279

Histopathology of psoriasis The microscopic picture of typical psoriasis is generally diagnostic. In Fig. 278, one sees a markedly thickened stratum corneum with retained nuclei (parakeratosis) and focal collections of degenerating neutrophils (microabscesses of Munro). The stratum granulosum has disappeared, and the rete ridges of the stratum malpighii are fairly uniform in length, club-shaped, and fused. The interdigitating dermal papillae reach very close to the surface, with thinning of the overlying epidermal suprapapillary plates.

Often the papillae contain prominent, thin-walled blood vessels, which easily rupture when the surface scale is forcibly removed, resulting in minute bleeding points (Auspitz sign). In the migration of neutrophils toward the stratum corneum, as they seem to be released in intermittent bursts from the papillary vessels, accumulations of them may develop high in the malpighian layer, producing the so-called spongiform pustule of Kogoj, one of which is seen in Fig. 279.

Figure 280

Figure 281

Psoriasis (cont.) Psoriasis of the nail plates is a frequent manifestation of the disease and exceedingly difficult to treat. The most characteristic and often the earliest change is the formation of numerous small pits in the surface of the nail plate. As the disease progresses, the nail becomes discolored, and there is subungual hyperkeratosis, onycholysis (separation of nail bed and nail plate), and onychomadesis (shedding). Figure 280 illustrates severe involvement with crumbling in two fingernails and minimal disease in the nails of the neighboring fingers. Figure 281 illustrates generalized psoriasis. Almost the entire body is covered with scaly lesions. Some such cases also go on to exfoliative erythroderma. The condition then is not only disfiguring and uncomfortable but is severely disruptive to cutaneous function. Problems arise with respect to heat regulation, sweating, and maintenance of electrolyte balance. Protein loss from excessive scaling is metabolically disruptive. Hospitalization and careful management of this condition are required.

Figure 282

Figure 283

Psoriasis These figures illustrate pustular psoriasis. Both are examples of the disease in relatively mild form, but even in these the suppurative quality of the lesions can be appreciated. Severe pustular psoriasis, also known as the von Zumbusch form, is a rare and potentially life-threatening disease. Pustular psoriasis may be triggered by physical or emotional stress, a number of medications, or the abrupt discontinuation of steroid therapy. Patients with this disease form develop shaking chills, fever, and leukocytosis. Numerous superficial pustules develop on psoriatic plaques and on uninvolved skin. Over a brief period of time, the pustules enlarge and become confluent; lakes of pus form. The process may eventuate in an exfoliative erythroderma. Hospitalization and careful supportive therapy are important aspects of treatment.

Figure 284

Figure 285

Pityriasis rubra pilaris This is a chronic and often severe cutaneous disorder that may sometimes begin during childhood. Depending on the stage and location of the disease process, the appearance varies. The most unique manifestation of this disease are the red-orange perifollicular keratotic papules that are usually located on the dorsum of the fingers and hands. The "nutmeg grater" appearance in these areas is virtually pathognomonic of pityriasis rubra pilaris. Figures

284 and 285 illustrate the disease process as it appears on the trunk. Here, follicular localization may be apparent early in the condition, but later, plaques of scaling, erythema, and edema are more usual. The condition may become generalized, but usually some islands of normal-appearing skin remain interspersed between involved areas. A similar erythema and scaling of the face and scalp may represent the initial presentation of pityriasis rubra pilaris.

Figure 286

Figure 287

Pityriasis rubra pilaris Figure 286 shows both discrete follicular papules and larger confluent, psoriasiform plaques on the leg. Palmoplantar involvement in pityriasis rubra pilaris is very common and can be disabling. Figure 287 pictures the highly characteristic appearance of the condition on the palms. There is a diffuse hyperkeratosis that is symmetrical and covers the entire palmar surface. Similar changes may be present on the soles of the feet, and dystrophy of both fingernails and toenails may be prominent. Pityriasis rubra

pilaris in children has been divided into subtypes based on natural history and clinical appearance. The *classic* juvenile form affects children in the first 2 years of life and often tends to become generalized and severe. The *circumscribed* juvenile type presents with patches of follicular papules and displays a lesser tendency toward progression to generalized disease. Finally, the *atypical* juvenile form is the rarest, has the poorest prognosis, and tends to be familial.

Figure 288

Figure 289

Pityriasis rosea　This benign and self-limited eruption occurs most often in the spring and autumn. Most patients are adolescents and young adults, but the disorder is not unusual in children and may even occur during infancy. In its classic form, pityriasis rosea follows a specific and predictable clinical course. The first, solitary lesion is a circle or oval of erythema and scaling. As it develops to its full size of 2–3 cm, this so-called herald patch may easily be mistaken for a lesion of tinea corporis. The chest and upper thigh are a common location for the herald patch, but any area may be involved.

A typical herald patch is shown in Fig. 288. Within a period of 5–15 days, additional lesions begin to develop. Patients develop numerous round-to-oval pink-orange macules that are 3–10 mm in diameter. Each has an edge of fine scaling, the characteristic "collarette." Larger, round-to-oval patches may also be present. The lesions of pityriasis rosea tend to cluster on the trunk and proximal extremities and often are most numerous in the axillae. The generalized process is illustrated in Fig. 289. The duration of the total process is 6–9 weeks.

Figure 290

Figure 291

Pityriasis rosea　These figures illustrate well-developed lesions of pityriasis rosea in the mid-course of the condition. In Fig. 290, the fine rim of scale on the periphery of each lesion may be noted. In addition, one can appreciate the parallel array of the individual macules. On the back and chest, this tendency of the lesions to follow skin lines (the so-called Christmas tree distribution) is usually most obvious. A number of atypical forms of pityriasis may occur, and these variations in both morphology and distribution seem to

be more common during childhood. In particular, papules, pustules, and even vesicles may occur and their presence may suggest a number of other cutaneous disorders. However, a careful search will usually lead to one or several of the typical papulosquamous lesions. In addition, lesions may extend to involve the face and there may be relative sparing of the trunk. In some cases, the process is entirely intertriginous.

Figure 292

Figure 293

Guttate parapsoriasis (pityriasis lichenoides chronica) The term *parapsoriasis* is used to describe a number of unrelated dermatologic conditions which are also unrelated to psoriasis. Guttate parapsoriasis is a chronic disorder which is relatively unusual in children. It consists of superficial lesions which evolve from papules into oval, pink-brown papulosquamous lesions. There may be an adherent scale overlying the individual lesions, and there is sometimes mild pruritus. Involvement tends to favor the trunk and proximal extremi-

ties, although it may become more widespread. Many cases of guttate parapsoriasis are initially diagnosed as pityriasis rosea. However, the persistent course of this disease, with remissions and exacerbations, eventually distinguishes it. A number of treatment modalities have been tried, but none has been consistently successful. Guttate parapsoriasis has no systemic manifestations and must not be confused with a similar-sounding, unrelated condition, large plaque parapsoriasis, a form of mycosis fungoides.

Figure 294

Figure 295

Pityriasis lichenoides et varioliformis acuta (PLEVA, Mucha-Habermann disease) This is a troubling papulosquamous disorder of acute onset that occurs in both children and young adults. The individual lesions go though a distinctive process of evolution over a period of weeks. Each begins as an erythematous papule. The lesion enlarges to a brownish 2–3 mm oval and then develops a central area of vesiculation or a hemorrhagic or necrotic crust. Lesions of this type are depicted in both photographs. Involvement tends to favor the anterior trunk and proximal extremities. The axilla, as in

Fig. 294, is a particularly common location. Facial and palm and sole involvement is relatively rare, and pruritus is usually absent. The condition has no systemic manifestations and tends to improve gradually over a period of 4–6 months. However, some childhood cases last considerably longer, and scarring and pigmentary changes frequently occur. It appears that the resolution of this process can be hastened by a course of oral erythromycin. The mechanism of action of the drug in this situation is not known.

Figure 296

Figure 297

Lichen planus This condition is a pruritic eruption of un-known etiology. It is not uncommon in childhood. These illustrations are of the most representative lesions of lichen planus on a most common site, the wrists. The primary lesion consists of a flat-topped, polygonal, violaceous papule 2–6 mm in diameter. The characteristic shiny appearance of the individual papules is seen best in Fig. 297. The same figure illustrates the tendency for the solitary lesions to form confluent plaques. Exaggerated surface markings in the over-

lying skin (Wickham's striae) may also be evident but are difficult to appreciate from these photographs. The forearms, the middle of the back, and the anterior surfaces of the lower extremities are other common locations. On the legs, lesions may become markedly hypertrophic and plaque-like. Diag-nosis can sometimes be confirmed by the presence of oral lesions. Typically, there are small white papules in a reticular pattern on the buccal mucosa. The tongue, lips, and palate may also be involved.

Figure 298

Figure 299

Lichen planus The clinical severity of lichen planus varies from a few, mildly pruritic lesions in some cases, to extensive and severe involvement of the skin and mucous membranes with intractable itching in others. The latter situation is illustrated in Fig. 298. Children with limited disease often respond well to the local application of topical corticosteroids. However, when the process is generalized, a short course of systemic steroids may be necessary and will sometimes yield

a dramatic improvement. Lichen planus tends to be a problem of long duration, with periods of remission and exacerbation. Figure 299 illustrates the tendency for new lesions to form in a scratch or abrasion. The so-called Koebner phenomenon is highly characteristic of lichen planus, and some evidence of "Koebnerization" is seen in almost every patient with this disorder.

Figure 300

Figure 301

Lichen planus Most often, the lesions of lichen planus are small purplish papules, solitary or confluent, with exaggerated surface markings. There are, however, several variants. Some lesions develop adherent scales, sometimes vesiculation occurs, and, rarely, necrosis and scarring may occur upon resolution. The lesions in Fig. 300 are larger and more inflammatory than usual; there is a suggestion of vesiculation and necrosis. The vesicular and bullous forms of lichen planus must sometimes be differentiated from other bullous disorders. Figure 301, closely examined, shows a suggestion of scaling. Although the etiology of lichen planus remains a mystery, the clinician must bear in mind that certain lichenoid drug eruptions may be clinically indistinguishable from true lichen planus. The most common agents are gold salts and antimalarials. Topical exposure to paraphenylenediamine may have the same result.

Figure 302

Figure 303

Lichen planus A small percentage of patients with lichen planus develop nail involvement. The severity varies. Some children develop only mild thinning or ridging of the nail plate. Others have a severe nail dystrophy, with pterygium formation and complete and permanent nail loss. A case where the nails are destroyed is pictured here. Rarely, there may even be severe lichen planus of the fingernails and toenails without skin involvement. In any case, attempts to treat the severe forms of nail disease in lichen planus are rarely successful.

Histopathology of lichen planus Typical cases of lichen planus are clinically and histologically distinctive. Microscopically one sees the stratum corneum to be hyperkeratotic (not parakeratotic), overlying a stratum granulosum that is thickened. The entire epidermis (suprapapillary plates and rete ridges) is hyperplastic in a plate-like manner. The dermoepidermal interface is blurred by a subepidermal band of mononuclear inflammatory cells.

Figure 304

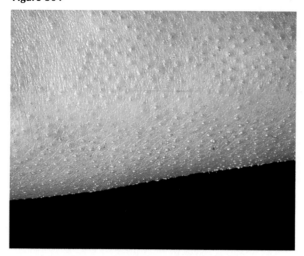

Lichen planopilaris (follicular lichen planus) This is a variant of lichen planus in which the primary involvement occurs around hair follicles. It is more common in women. Patients with this form of disease are also likely to have the more typical flat-topped papules and mucosal lesions as well. Pictured here are numerous, rough follicular papules on an extremity. Lichen planopilaris can be a severe and disfiguring disorder when it involves the scalp. In such cases, either a temporary or permanent, scarring alopecia may develop.

Figure 305

Lichen nitidus This is an unusual and distinctive dermatosis that has its peak incidence during childhood. The individual papules, as pictured here, are smaller than 1 mm in diameter. They are flat and shiny, with a round or polygonal shape. The lesions usually cluster, and an occasional linear grouping suggests that they occur in areas of trauma (the Koebner phenomenon). Lichen nitidus is occasionally seen in association with lichen planus. However, the marked differences in both histopathology and natural history indicate that they are different diseases.

Figure 306

Lichen nitidus In this illustration, the shiny character of the lesions of lichen nitidus is more appreciable. The penis is a site of predilection for this condition, as are the abdomen and upper extremities. The lesions of lichen nitidus are usually asymptomatic, but pruritus may occur. They may clear spontaneously in a short period of time, or they may last for months or years. There is no known effective treatment for the condition itself; itching can be treated symptomatically with antihistamines and mild topical steroids.

Figure 307

Histopathology of lichen nitidus Lichen nitidus is an uncommon dermatosis that has many clinical and histologic similarities to lichen planus. Fine differences are, however, what distinguish it. Microscopically, the thickened stratum corneum is parakeratotic; the stratum granulosum is gone; the stratum malpighii is thinned. A band-like infiltrate of cells hugs the overlying epidermis, but it is discontinuous and is somewhat granulomatous, as can be judged from the giant cell on the left.

Figure 308

Figure 309

Darier's disease (keratosis follicularis) This autosomal dominant disorder usually begins during mid-childhood. The primary lesion is a small crusted papule; in some areas these coalesce to form hyperkeratotic, greasy plaques. The lesions tend to favor so-called seborrheic areas, and the upper back and chest, as shown in Fig. 308, are the most common locations. In more severe cases there is extensive scalp and facial involvement, and there are moist, erythematous vegetating plaques in the flexures (Fig. 309). Small warty papules on the dorsum of the hands are a common finding. The lesions

tend to worsen in the summer; both humidity and ultraviolet light have a negative effect on the disease process. Nail involvement is characteristic of Darier's disease and may include red or white longitudinal streaks, thinning or thickening of the nail plate, and subungual hyperkeratosis. The severity of Darier's disease differs greatly among members of the same affected family. The use of synthetic retinoids in the most severe cases must be balanced against the problems of long-term toxicity.

Figure 310

Figure 311

Histopathology of Darier's disease (keratosis follicularis) *Keratosis follicularis* is a misnomer because the lesions are not exclusively follicular. The stratum corneum is thickened, elevated above the adjacent surface, and invaginated to form a plug. In the latter, one finds keratinized cells (grains) and large round cells with clear halos (corps ronds). The subjacent stratum malpighii is acanthotic, usually papillomatous, and marked by slits (lacunae).

Infundibulofolliculitis The intraepidermal portion of the pilosebaceous apparatus is called the infundibulum. In microscopy its vaguely funnel shape can be appreciated. Inflammation of the hair follicle at different levels and by different causes, microbial or inanimate, produces different pictures. At the level of the hair bulb, abscesses or furuncles are the usual lesions; above that level, pustules develop; and still higher, about the infundibulum, inflammatory papules (as pictured) are the lesions.

Figure 312

Figure 313

Lichen spinulosus   This condition consists of a small aggregation of keratotic papules at the openings of the hair follicles. The follicular hyperkeratosis is so marked that the involved area has an appreciable spiny texture. The typical circular or oval plaque is present in Fig. 312. The same process in a

more linear arrangement is shown in Fig. 313. Lichen spinulosus is probably most common among children with atopic dermatitis. Effective treatment may be achieved by use of topical preparations containing keratolytics, such as small percentages of salicylic acid (2–3%) and urea (10–20%).

Figure 314

Figure 315

Perforating folliculitis   This eruption consists of numerous small erythematous follicular papules with central keratotic plugging. The lesions, which vary in size from 2 to 8 mm., are usually located on the buttocks and thighs. The cause of this eruption is unknown; irritation of the hair follicle is probably the primary process. At various times, perforating folliculitis has been ascribed to the wearing of tight garments or to some chemical in clothing.

Histopathology of perforating folliculitis   In contrast to types of folliculitis that are acute inflammatory processes, perforating folliculitis is a disorder of keratinization. A plug of horn, together with some basophilic debris, is seen within the distended upper portion of a pilosebaceous unit. The follicular epithelium is thinned almost to nothing at the lower left edge of the plug, and the surrounding connective tissue is but moderately inflamed.

Figure 316

Reactive perforating collagenosis This rare autosomal recessive disease usually has its onset during infancy and early childhood. The lesions, as shown here, consist of small erythematous papules that gradually increase in size and develop a central hyperkeratotic plug. In some cases, the linear array of lesions suggests that they are induced by trauma—the so-called Koebner phenomenon. Pruritus is an occasional feature. Lesions usually last 6–8 weeks and then resolve, only to be followed by the eruption of fresh papules.

Figure 317

Histopathology of reactive perforating collagenosis This rare condition is secondary to trauma of a kind that damages collagen in localized areas in the upper cutis. The injured collagen is slowly extruded to the surface by a process of transepithelial elimination, often with scarring. During the active stage, a plug of horn and debris, at times a crust, forms on the surface and sits in a cup-shaped depression of the subjacent epidermis. Mild dermal inflammation is present.

Figure 318

Follicular mucinosis (alopecia mucinosa) This is an uncommon disorder of unknown etiology which affects both children and adults. The lesions, which are usually located on the head and neck, vary in clinical appearance. Most often, as illustrated here, there are grouped flesh-colored papules. There may also be erythematous plaques with follicular accentuation and scale. When the disorder affects the scalp, it causes areas of permanent alopecia. In children, this disease tends to resolve spontaneously. However, an association with lymphoma may rarely occur.

Figure 319

Histopathology of follicular mucinosis Follicular mucinosis (alopecia mucinosa), as it occurs in children, is usually a self-limited disease. The pilosebaceous unit is not destroyed but assumes an edematous or even cystic appearance by accumulation of acid mucopolysaccharide (mainly hyaluronic acid), which here stains blue against a pink background. Digestion with testicular hyaluronidase eliminates the positive staining.

Figure 320

Figure 321

Porokeratosis (porokeratosis of Mibelli) This is a rare autosomal dominant dermatosis with unique clinical and histologic findings. Lesions usually develop during childhood and favor the hands, forearms, and face. Each individual lesion begins as a papule and evolves into an irregular atrophic plaque. A well-developed plaque is pictured in Fig. 320. The elevated and hyperpigmented border, with a fine groove running throughout, is somewhat difficult to appreciate in this photograph. This border, which corresponds to the histologic

cornoid lamella, is the most diagnostic clinical feature. Note the two lesions in Fig. 321. Here one can begin to appreciate the raised hyperkeratotic border which surrounds each circinate plaque. In some cases, lesions are arranged in a linear array. There are two other forms of porokeratosis: the disseminated superficial actinic type (numerous small lesions on sun-exposed skin) and porokeratosis palmaris et plantaris disseminata (an autosomal dominant syndrome which begins on the palms and soles).

Figure 322

Histopathology of porokeratosis The classic condition develops in childhood or early adult life, usually as a ringed lesion, the elevated margin of which constitutes the active area where the biopsy is best taken. That margin consists of a vertical or oblique column of thickened parakeratotic horn (the cornoid lamella) seated in a small depression of hyperplastic stratum malpighii. At the base of the cornoid lamella the stratum granulosum is attenuated or absent.

Figure 323

Figure 324

Elastosis perforans serpiginosa This rare disorder is characterized by small cone-shaped hyperkeratotic papules that are arranged in annular or circinate patterns. The lesions are usually localized; involvement in two common locations, the side of the face and the nape of the neck, is illustrated here. The process may also be disseminated. The underlying histologic process is the transepidermal elimination of elastic tissue. An association with heritable disorders such as Ehlers-

Danlos syndrome, Marfan syndrome, pseudoxanthoma elasticum, osteogenesis imperfecta, Rothmund-Thomson syndrome, and Down's syndrome has been reported. Elastosis perforans serpiginosa may also occur as a side effect of treatment with penicillamine. In most patients, there is no effective therapy. Attempts at surgical removal are complicated by the high incidence of recurrence and scar formation.

Figure 325

Histopathology of elastosis perforans serpiginosa This condition may resemble porokeratosis clinically when both have ringed lesions with elevated borders. Microscopically in elastosis perforans serpiginosa, hyperplasia of elastic fibers develops in the papillae. Some of the elastica is eliminated by transepithelial expulsion. In this photomicrograph, one sees within an acanthotic stratum malpighii three masses of degenerating elastic tissue and debris en route to the surface.

10

Nutritional and Metabolic Disorders

Figure 326

Figure 327

Acrodermatitis enteropathica   The four pictures on this page show the major cutaneous manifestations of acrodermatitis enteropathica. This syndrome results from inadequate dietary intake or absorption of zinc. Figure 326 shows erythema, crusting, and fissuring of the perioral skin and cheeks. The eruption that is pictured here may be preceded by blisters. The diaper area in Fig. 327 is diffusely erythematous and has a sharply marginated border on the abdomen. Other features of acrodermatitis enteropathica include stomatitis, parony-

chia, and alopecia. Acrodermatitis enteropathica may be inherited in autosomal recessive fashion. This form of the disease seems to be related to an inability to absorb zinc. Acquired acrodermatitis enteropathica is seen in infants who have received parenteral alimentation lacking sufficient zinc and, rarely, in breast-fed premature infants who have larger dietary zinc requirements. Occasionally, acrodermatitis enteropathica in a full-term breast-fed infant may be the result of low levels of zinc in the breast milk.

Figure 328

Figure 329

Acrodermatitis enteropathica   Figure 328 shows a highly characteristic picture of the cutaneous changes of acrodermatitis enteropathica about the anus, buttocks, and on the perineum. Note how psoriasiform this lesion and those on the feet in Fig. 329 are. The full-blown picture of acrodermatitis enteropathica goes far beyond the typical changes of skin and hair. Affected children have severe diarrhea, growth retardation, and irritability. Without treatment, the disease

follows a progressive course and may even be fatal. The crucial relationship between acrodermatitis enteropathica and zinc deficiency was discovered in 1973. The child with suspected acrodermatitis enteropathica should be evaluated for a low serum zinc level. (Blood must be drawn in plastic non-rubber stoppered tubes to avoid the possibility of zinc contamination.) Treatment with dietary zinc supplementation leads to a dramatic resolution of all symptoms.

Figure 330

Figure 331

Cutaneous expressions of kwashiorkor Kwashiorkor is a type of protein energy malnutrition. It is seen most commonly in developing countries, and onset tends to occur after weaning. At that time, the balance of protein and carbohydrate in breast milk is replaced by a diet that contains almost exclusively carbohydrates. The initial signs are diarrhea, irritability, and edema of the hands and feet. Small dark patches appear at pressure points of the elbows, ankles, wrists, and knees, which then spread. The patches have a sharp border and tend to peel; the superficial desquamation in these areas is often likened to the appearance of flaking paint or enamel. As the condition progresses, there develops a generalized red-brown discoloration. Other findings include fissuring at the edges of the mouth (Fig. 330) and the development of coarse, hypopigmented hair. Photosensitivity and easy bruising may also be present. The child with severe kwashiorkor appears extremely apathetic and has generalized edema. Pictured in Fig. 331 is a child with areas of desquamation and anasarca. Kwashiorkor carries a high mortality rate. With timely dietary intervention, it can often be reversed.

Figure 332

Figure 333

Cutaneous expressions of pellagra Pellagra is a disease caused by inadequate dietary intake of niacin. It is now seen in parts of the world where dietary intake of tryptophan, an amino acid precursor of niacin, is inadequate. In particular, diets which consist largely or exclusively of maize or millet predispose to this disease. The signs and symptoms of pellagra are often remembered by the mnemonic four Ds: dermatitis, diarrhea, dementia, and death. The classic cutaneous changes are inflammation, hyperpigmentation, and scaling in symmetric distribution and in areas exposed to heat or sunlight. Typical areas of involvement are the hands and forearms, legs and feet, and face and neck. Figure 332 shows moderate changes on the feet and legs. Figure 333 shows the scaling dermatitis on the face and an angular cheilitis. Edema and inflammation of the tongue are also common features of pellagra. The addition of supplemental niacin to the diet brings a quick resolution to the disease.

Figure 334

Figure 335

Cutaneous expressions of phenylketonuria This is a rare metabolic disorder that is inherited in autosomal recessive fashion. Children with the disease have a defect in the enzyme phenylalanine hydroxylase and are unable to convert phenylalanine to tyrosine. There are several associated cutaneous changes. Affected individuals have fairer skin and lighter-colored hair than their normal siblings; Caucasians with the disease typically have blond hair and blue eyes. Because the melanocytes of patients with phenylketonuria are less able to manufacture melanin, patients tend to sunburn easily. In addition, an eczematous dermatitis is a common component of phenylketonuria. The lesions may resemble atopic dermatitis in morphology and distribution, as in these figures. In other patients, the dermatitis is more widespread. Treatment of this disease consists of dietary restriction of phenylalanine. The early institution of this diet limits the possibility of severe intellectual impairment, which is the most significant aspect of the disease.

Figure 336

Figure 337

Cutaneous expressions of erythropoietic protoporphyria This is among the more common porphyrias; onset is usually during early childhood. The typical presentation of this disease features the development of pruritus and burning of the skin in areas of recent sun exposure. These sensations may be accompanied by erythema, edema, and vesiculation. Over time, superficial scarring and a waxy thickening of the involved areas develop. These changes, as seen on the hands and feet, are illustrated here. The bridge of the nose is another common area of involvement. Children with erythropoietic protoporphyria have inherited a deficiency of the enzyme ferrochelatase, which normally converts protoporphyrin to heme. The disease can be readily diagnosed by the combination of the clinical findings outlined above and an elevated free erythrocyte protoporphyrin level. The most serious complication is the development of hepatic involvement. Treatment of the skin disease consists of avoidance of the sun and oral therapy with beta-carotene.

Figure 338

Figure 339

Lipoid proteinosis (hyalinosis cutis et mucosae) This is a rare autosomal recessive disease which is caused by the deposition of hyaline material in the skin and mucous membranes. Laryngeal involvement may be present from birth and eventually produces a characteristic hoarseness in every affected individual. Cutaneous disease begins during the first 2 years of life and consists of papules, nodules, and areas of

thickening and hyperkeratosis. The cutaneous lesions on the alae nasi and in the choanae are shown in Fig. 338. In Fig. 339, the mucosal surface of the lower lip is extensively involved with the characteristic papules. Not shown here are the numerous small papules which dot the free margins of the eyelids. The disorder is attributed to a defect in glycoprotein metabolism, but the exact mechanism is unknown.

Figure 340

Figure 341

Lipoid proteinosis Pictured here are a plaque and lesions of smaller sizes on and around the elbow. Most patients with lipoid proteinosis continue to develop additional lesions during adult life. The most serious sequelae are caused by lesions in the mouth and oropharynx. The tongue may become thick and bound down, and dysphagia and respiratory obstruction may result from lesions in the pharynx and larynx. Finally, intracranial calcifications are a common feature of lipoid proteinosis. For most patients these are asymptomatic, but seizure disorders may occur.

Hurler's syndrome This inherited condition results in the accumulation of chondroitin sulfate B in the skin and other organ systems. Dwarfism and an unusual facial appearance are also aspects of the disease. This photograph is an excellent representation of shagreen skin, an appearance that is also seen in tuberous sclerosis. *Shagreen* refers to a type of leather that is embossed with knobs by processing and then variably stained.

Figure 342

Xanthomatosis Xanthomas are papules or nodules of the skin or mucous membranes that contain lipids. The appearance of xanthomas during childhood should trigger a thorough search for underlying systemic disease. The yellowish papules in Fig. 342 are a form of planar xanthoma. These may occur on any part of the body and may be an indicator of a hereditary lipoproteinemia, diabetes mellitus, or liver disease. Multiple myeloma and histiocytosis X are less common etiologies. The patient pictured here has biliary cirrhosis.

Figure 343

Xanthomatosis The lesions illustrated here are typical of xanthoma striatum palmare, a form of planar xanthoma. This patient also has biliary cirrhosis. Note how the yellowish papules and plaques follow the creases of the fingers and the palmar folds. The familial hyperlipidemias, particularly types II, III and V, may present with the identical clinical picture. Patients with these disorders are at high risk for ischemic heart disease.

Figure 344

Xanthomatosis These small papules on the dorsum of the feet are also xanthomas. The patient is a 4-year-old child with type II hyperlipoproteinemia. This is an autosomal dominant condition in which there may be massive elevations in serum cholesterol. Individuals with this disease often develop ischemic heart disease during young adulthood. The recognition of the cutaneous lesions is important in identifying children who may require dietary or medical management of their hypercholesterolemia.

Figure 345

Xanthomatosis These yellow-red nodules, which often occur on the elbows and knees, are termed *tuberous xanthomas*. They may also be found on other areas where ordinary trauma is common, e.g., buttocks, knuckles, and heels. Similar lesions which overlie extensor tendons are sometimes called *tendon xanthomas*. Lesions of this sort are almost always caused by a hyperlipoproteinemia and should prompt investigation of serum cholesterol and triglycerides. Types II, IV, and V are the ones that are most commonly associated with tuberous and tendon xanthomas.

Figure 346

Xanthomatosis Not all xanthomatoses are rooted in abnormalities of cholesterol metabolism or other systemic disease. In this illustration, xanthomatous papules that developed in a lymphedematous leg are shown. Since serum lipids are normal, local causes stemming from the lymphatic obstruction must account for the lesions. The condition does not have the serious import of those xanthomatoses associated with abnormalities of serum lipids.

Figure 347

Calcinosis cutis When calcification occurs in the skin, it may represent either an isolated local event, or it may be a sign of an underlying systemic disease. The lesion pictured here is a solitary nodular calcification. These sometimes result from local trauma, such as an insect bite, or from the rupture of an epidermal cyst (dystrophic calcinosis cutis). When such nodules occur on the face of an infant they are usually idiopathic and of no medical significance.

Figure 348

Calcinosis cutis The nodular calcifications pictured here also turned out to be idiopathic. However, grouped calcifications like these may also be seen in children with CRST syndrome (calcinosis cutis, Raynaud's phenomenon, sclerodactyly, telangiectasia) or dermatomyositis. Pseuodxanthoma elasticum and Ehlers-Danlos syndrome are other causes. So-called metastatic calcinosis cutis, with widespread precipitation of calcium salts, is a sign of abnormal calcium metabolism and may result from parathyroid tumors, chronic renal failure, or vitamin D intoxication.

Figure 349

Histopathology of calcinosis cutis Insoluble salts of calcium may be deposited ectopically in soft tissues (in skin uncommonly) as a result of obviously deranged calcium-phosphorus metabolism (in parathyroidism, renal disease, etc.), following trauma (ossifying myositis), in association with abnormal or altered tissue (scleroderma), and for no apparent reason. Such is the case illustrated. Calcium salts are seen as amorphous basophilic material surrounded by a pronounced cellular response.

11

Genodermatoses

Figure 350

Figure 351

Pseudoxanthoma elasticum This is a generalized condition in which elastic fibers are degenerative. Clinical signs of the phenomenon can be recognized in the skin and eyes. In the skin, patches of yellowish discoloration and general laxness or redundancy develop on the neck ("chicken skin"), in the axillae, and in other places like the fossae of limbs and the inguinal folds where considerable movement of skin is normal. In the eye, so-called angioid streaks can be seen. They represent the result of faulty elastic fibers in Bruch's mem-

brane and generally precede the cutaneous changes. These eye changes frequently result in the loss of central vision and sometimes result in blindness. Gastrointestinal hemorrhage is the most serious acute consequence, but slower structural damage in various organs may result in hypertension, coronary artery occlusion, diabetes mellitus, thyroid dyscrasia, or ectopic calcinosis. The disease may be inherited in autosomal recessive or autosomal dominant fashion.

Figure 352

Figure 353

Histopathology of pseudoxanthoma elasticum The diagnosis of pseudoxanthoma elasticum is confirmable by biopsy. The elastic fibers of the midcutis are abnormal both morphologically and tinctorially. This is easily appreciated with this stain for elastic tissue. The slightly wavy fibers high in the photomicrograph are normal; the deeper fibers are disrupted and granular. When stained with hematoxylin and eosin, they are basophilic, indicating calcification.

Cutis laxa In this condition, elastic fibers are decreased in number by an unknown mechanism. As seen in this patient, the skin hangs in folds and produces an appearance of premature aging. Because elastic fibers are affected in all organ systems, intestinal and urinary bladder diverticulae, rectal prolapse, inguinal hernias, and pulmonary emphysema frequently occur. The last of these is associated with significant mortality. The most common and severe form is inherited in autosomal recessive fashion.

Figure 354

Figure 355

The Ehlers-Danlos syndrome This syndrome is actually a collection of 11 discrete conditions with the common features of hyperextensible skin and joints, easy bruising, defective wound healing, and blood vessel fragility. Distinct abnormalities in collagen synthesis have been identified in some of the varieties of Ehlers-Danlos syndrome. The result of the anomaly is extreme stretchability but unimpaired elasticity (i.e., the ability to return to normal after stretching). The photographs illustrate the phenomenon; Figure 354 shows

skin of the neck and Fig. 355 of the elbow extended several times more than normal skin can be pulled out. Depending on the type, inheritance may be autosomal dominant, autosomal recessive, or X-linked recessive. Gastrointestinal perforation and rupture of a large artery are the most severe complications of this syndrome. Premature birth (probably due to fragility of the fetal membranes) is a common event in patients with Ehlers-Danlos.

Figure 356

Figure 357

The Ehlers-Danlos syndrome In these illustrations more of the hyperextensible phenomena and the consequences of functional abnormality of elastic fibers and collagen are shown. Figure 356 shows hyperextensibility of joints, from which it may be inferred that skin, ligament, tendon, and to some extent bone are abnormally stretchable. Another way in which softness of muscle and related structures can be appreciated is the feel of a handshake with a patient who has the Ehlers-Danlos syndrome. No matter how hard one presses,

there is a feeling that one is not quite through with the handshake, so compressible is the hand. Figure 357 illustrates the result of incisions and shearing trauma in the skin of a patient with the Ehlers-Danlos syndrome. The result is hemorrhage, failure of healing by primary intention, and finally broad, friable scars. Small "pseudotumors" on the elbows and knees are actually calcified herniations of fat through the dermis.

Figure 358

Figure 359

Focal dermal hypoplasia   This is a combination of disordered structure of ectodermal and mesenchymal tissue of both skin and bone. The most common cutaneous lesions are linear or reticulate areas of hypoplasia with telangiectasia, atrophy, and abnormal pigmentation. Figure 358 shows some such patches, and the nodular fat tumors which are typically present. Figure 359 illustrates the frequent involvement of the perioral skin and teeth. Papillomas may also be present within the mouth. Many affected individuals have dysplastic or absent fingernails and toenails and patches of alopecia. The range of clinical possibilities may be from minor process on the limbs to extensive distortion of the skin and bony skeleton. When bone is involved, syndactyly, adactyly, skeletal asymmetry, and scoliosis may occur. Ocular abnormalities include colobomas, microphthalmia, and strabismus. A variety of genetic mechanisms have been suggested to explain the fact that 90 percent of patients are female.

Figure 360

Figure 361

Histopathology of focal dermal hypoplasia   Of the many abnormalities in this complex syndrome, the histologically specific one is almost total absence of dermis. In the photomicrograph one sees the adipose tissue, which normally is limited to the subcutis, lying under the epidermis, separated from it by an almost imperceptible bit of connective tissue. A similar picture may be seen in nevus lipomatosus, which, however, can be distinguished clinically.

Cutaneous expressions of the Wiskott-Aldrich syndrome   This is another severe immunologic defect with X-linked recessive inheritance. The classic symptoms of this disease, which occurs only in males, are thrombocytopenia, recurrent infection, and a generalized eczematous or exfoliative dermatitis. Children with this disorder have impaired humoral and cell-mediated immunity, with deficient IgM and elevated IgA, and are at risk for sepsis and hemorrhage. The figure shows the kind of petechiae that are evidence of the persistent thrombocytopenia.

Figure 362

Figure 363

Cutaneous expressions of ataxia telangiectasia   This autosomal recessive disorder affects the skin and the immunologic and central nervous systems. The onset of the disease, during early childhood, is characterized by the combination of progressive cerebellar ataxia and telangiectasias. The earliest site of telangiectasia is usually the bulbar conjunctiva, as pictured in Fig. 362. These vascular lesions also involve the neck, upper chest, face, and, as illustrated in Fig. 363, the pinna of the ear. Later cutaneous changes include blotchy

hyper- and hypopigmentation, café-au-lait spots, hirsutism, and a generalized eczematous dermatitis. There may be premature graying of the hair. The immunologic abnormalities include decreased levels of IgA and IgE and defective cell-mediated immunity. Children with ataxia telangiectasia suffer from recurrent sinopulmonary infection and may die from bronchiectasis and respiratory failure. Lymphoreticular malignancies are an additional complication.

Figure 364

Figure 365

Cutaneous expressions of Bloom's syndrome   The principle cutaneous manifestations of this autosomal recessive syndrome are erythema and telangiectasias of the cheeks and photosensitivity. Café-au-lait spots and acanthosis nigricans may also be present. Children with Bloom's syndrome are small at birth and have severe growth retardation throughout life. They also have recurrent respiratory infections and a strong tendency to develop malignancy. This rare disease is attributed to chromosomal abnormalities and defects in DNA repair. Chromosome analysis is invariably abnormal.

Cutaneous expressions of poikiloderma congenitale (the Rothmund-Thomson syndrome)   This rare, inherited condition begins during infancy with typically progressive skin changes. Erythema and edema of the facial skin is rapidly followed by the development of atrophy and telangiectasia. The same process occurs on the buttocks and extremities. Cataracts develop in many patients, and these often become apparent during infancy or early childhood. Skeletal deformities and short stature are other occasional features of this disease.

Figure 366

Figure 367

Cutaneous expressions of Cockayne's syndrome   This is another rare autosomal recessive condition characterized by skin changes and dwarfism. During the second year of life, patients develop a scaly photoeruption on the face and upper neck. This resolves with hyperpigmentation. The scaling photodermatitis and typical bird-like facies of this syndrome are illustrated in Fig. 366. In addition to dwarfism (Fig. 367), affected individuals may demonstrate sensorineural deafness, microcephaly, and severe mental retardation. Optic atrophy and retinal degeneration may also be present. Characteristic intracranial calcifications are a feature of Cockayne's syndrome that may aid in confirmation of the diagnosis. The disorder has been attributed to a defect in DNA repair.

Figure 368

Figure 369

Congenital ectodermal dysplasia   Embryonic underdevelopment of the ectoderm is seen in two syndromes: anhidrotic and hidrotic ectodermal dysplasia. Figure 368 shows the faulty dentition and pathognomonic facies in the more severe anhidrotic type. This syndrome, which occurs almost exclusively in boys, may include alopecia, nail dystrophy, stunted growth, and severe mental retardation. Severe hyperthermia during warm weather is the result of the absence of normal perspiration, and therapy should be aimed at regulation of environmental temperature, decreased exercise, and cool clothing. The hidrotic type affects males and females equally and is generally less severe. There is no abnormal sweating. Dystrophic nails, which may be distorted in size, shape, color, or consistency, are the hallmark of the syndrome. Patients tend to have sparse body and scalp hair. The nail dystrophy may be accompanied by severe hyperkeratosis of the palms and soles, as seen in Fig. 369. Topical keratolytics are of some help to affected individuals.

Figure 370

Figure 371

Pachyonychia congenita This condition is a heritable syndrome in which there is severe dyskeratinization of a special sort that especially affects nails, palms and soles, and the mucous membranes of the lips and mouth. The nail changes are distinctive in their discoloration, hardness, excessive growth, and attachment to hyperkeratotic nail beds: Fig. 370 shows such nails, in which scleronychia and binding to the nail beds can be appreciated; Fig. 371 shows nails excessively

overgrown to the point of onychogryphosis. Not shown is hyperkeratotic process on palms and soles that can be as comparably bad as in nails. Nor is leukokeratosis of lips and tongue shown, a condition that severely disturbs function and is cosmetically distressing, to say the least. Aside from these major sites of hypertrophic dyskeratinization, there are other places and kinds of abnormality, which are shown below.

Figure 372

Figure 373

Pachyonychia congenita On the expanse of the body, especially on the buttocks and extremities, the dyskeratinization of pachyonychia congenita may take the form of what might be considered to be keratosis pilaris, except that forcible removal of the follicular keratotic plugs leaves cavities that have a tendency to bleed. This phenomenon is pictured in Fig. 372. More serious than follicular keratosis is a tendency to bulla formation on the lower part of the legs in a form that

suggests epidermolysis bullosa; Figure 373 shows how severe this part of the syndrome can be. Rooted as the entire condition is in a hereditary dyscrasia, there is no reasonable management of it. In the most severe instances of distortion of the nails, extirpation of the nail beds, even amputation of distal phalanges, may be required in order to achieve some degree of usable function of the fingers.

Figure 374

Figure 375

Dyskeratosis congenita This is another congenital and hereditary condition that is also rare, different from other dyskeratinizations, and distinctive. Its marks are skin changes in the form of atrophy and dyschromia, atrophic dysplasia of nails, and a kind of leukoplakia. In Fig. 374 those skin changes are shown as mottled or retiform poikiloderma. The face, neck, and upper part of the body are characteristically involved. The process goes on to fine atrophy and hypo- and

hyperpigmentation until the poikilodermatous character of the changes becomes established. The kind of process that occurs on mucous membranes is shown in Fig. 375. There are two lesions on the tongue that are gray and hypertrophic. The buccal mucosa and the mucosa of the urethra and anus may also be affected. Aside from the cutaneous and mucosal effects, abnormalities such as are seen in Fanconi's syndrome may be associated with this condition.

Figure 376

Figure 377

Dyskeratosis congenita Here are more possible cutaneous changes in dyskeratosis congenita: Fig. 376 shows hypoplastic nail changes that are characteristic. Note how different they are from those of pachyonychia congenita (Fig. 370). Instead of overgrowth, there is underdevelopment. Details of the cutaneous changes on glabrous skin in and about the groin are shown in Fig. 377. Note how similar they are to those on the neck and face. In addition to what has been illustrated,

hyperhidrosis of palms and soles, conjunctivitis, esophageal strictures, intestinal diverticula, mental retardation, and anemia may be parts of the syndrome. Malignant degeneration in the leukoplakia of the mucous membranes is a possibility. It is obvious that therapy for the condition is meager. Palliation of symptoms to whatever extent possible and observation for supervention of malignancy and the treatment thereof are all that can be done.

Figure 378

Figure 379

Neurofibromatosis (von Recklinghausen's disease) This autosomal dominant disorder includes a number of distinctive cutaneous findings and a wide variety of neurologic manifestations. Figure 378 shows a café-au-lait spot. Solitary lesions of this type are common in normal individuals; most patients with neurofibromatosis have more than a single macule. The presence of more than six lesions that are larger than 1.5 cm. in diameter is often considered to be a pathognomonic sign of the disease. In Fig. 379 there are several macules of hyperpigmentation in the axilla. Axillary freckling, also called

Crowe's sign, is a unique finding in neurofibromatosis. Pigmented hamartomas of the iris, termed *Lisch nodules,* are also present in almost all patients with this condition. The inheritance of neurofibromatosis is complicated by a very variable range of expression among those affected. A single family may include some individuals with only cutaneous involvement, and others with numerous neurofibromas or severe neurologic disease. Spontaneous mutations are also common.

Figure 380

Figure 381

Neurofibromatosis (von Recklinghausen's disease) These are more illustrations of the pigmentary anomalies and tumors in the skin of patients with neurofibromatosis; Figure 380 shows several café-au-lait spots and small tumors; Figure 381 shows a large café-au-lait spot on the left and a barely discernible tumor on the right. Neurofibromas have variable consistency. The soft lesions can be pushed into the surrounding skin, so-called buttonholing. Neurofibromas usually begin to develop during puberty and may cause severe cosmetic disfigurement.

Pruritus of the skin which overlies the neurofibroma is a common complaint, and the itching is aggravated by exertion or a warm environment. Malignant degeneration of a benign neurofibroma is a constant concern. In addition, patients with the disease are prone to develop neurofibrosarcomas or malignant schwannomas de novo. Selective surgical removal of neurofibromas, in order to improve either appearance or function, is feasible.

Figure 382

Figure 383

Neurofibromatosis (von Recklinghausen's disease) (cont.)
Figure 382 shows three café-au-lait spots and a small soft
neurofibroma. The enlargement in Fig. 383 was found to be
due to a neurofibroma in the palm and along the length of
the digits. Intellectual handicap, speech impediment, and
seizures are frequent manifestations of classic, or von Recklinghausen, neurofibromatosis. Although this form of neurofibromatosis tends to be progressive, it is entirely unpredictable. There is no single aspect of the clinical course which
allows the physician to foresee the evolution of other features.

Figure 384

Figure 385

Histopathology of neurofibromas Neurofibromas, whether
solitary or numerous (as in patients with von Recklinghausen's
disease), may show more or less histologic resemblance to
peripheral nerves, especially in deeper lesions obviously
related to nerves. Often the pattern is neuroid, at times
grossly plexiform. In most cutaneous lesions like the one
shown here, one merely sees cells with oval nuclei and
without plasma membranes, arranged randomly in a pink
fibrillar background.

Mucosal neuroma syndrome The presence of numerous
small neuromas of the lips, tongue, and oral mucosa is a
marker for a unique autosomal dominant condition. This
syndrome, now termed *multiple endocrine neoplasia type
2B*, carries a very high risk for malignancy. Eighty percent
of affected individuals will develop medullary thyroid carcinoma. Pheochromocytoma may also occur. This patient
developed both tumors, and had the marfanoid habitus that
is frequently seen in patients with the disorder.

Figure 386

Figure 387

Tuberous sclerosis This is an autosomal dominant disease with widely variable penetrance; its main effects are on the skin, central nervous system, eye, kidney, and heart. Figures 386 and 387 illustrate one of the most common cutaneous manifestations: adenoma sebaceum. The pink-to-red dome-shaped papules usually appear between the ages of 2 and 6. The lesions of adenoma sebaceum may be symmetrically distributed over the entire face but are usually most con-

centrated on the cheeks. Histologically, the individual papules are angiofibromas. The extent of cutaneous involvement is not generally predictive of the severity of the disease. Patients who are severely affected suffer from seizure disorders and mental retardation. Other findings of tuberous sclerosis include retinal and renal hamartomas, cerebral nodules and calcifications, and cardiac rhabdomyosarcomas.

Figure 388

Figure 389

Tuberous sclerosis Two cutaneous manifestations of the syndrome are shown in Fig. 388. Above and to the right is a hypopigmented macule, which sometimes takes the shape of an ash leaf. Hypopigmented macules may occur in healthy infants, but the appearance of several such lesions should trigger a search for other manifestations of tuberous sclerosis in the patient and family members. So-called ash leaf spots are the earliest cutaneous manifestation of the syndrome; they are either present at birth or evolve during infancy.

Wood's light examination may sometimes reveal hypopigmented macules whose presence is otherwise not obvious. In the midline in the same photograph is a shagreen patch, an area of cutaneous thickening with a pebbled surface. This lesion, frequently seen in children with tuberous sclerosis, is, histologically, a form of connective tissue nevus. In Fig. 389 there are subungual and periungual fibromas. These firm lesions arise from the nail beds, usually after puberty.

Figure 390

Figure 391

Basal cell nevus syndrome Patients with this autosomal dominant syndrome develop multiple basal cell carcinomas and cysts within the mandible. Additional findings include hypertelorism, a variety of other skeletal abnormalities, and calcification of the falx cerebri. Shown in Fig. 390 is an example of multiple basal cell carcinomas, which are unusually small in size. Most patients have more conventional lesions in the form of pearly telangiectatic nodules, sometimes with ulceration. Figure 391 shows the palmar pitting which appears during puberty in individuals with this syndrome. Rapidly enlarging basal cell carcinomas must be treated early on with the conventional surgical modalities in order to minimize disfigurement and avoid loss of function. Patients with basal cell nevus syndrome are also at risk for medulloblastoma. This grave complication tends to occur in early childhood.

Figure 392

Figure 393

Xeroderma pigmentosum This rare autosomal recessive disease is caused by an inability to repair DNA that has been damaged by ultraviolet light. There are at least eight different molecular defects. Freckling develops on sun-exposed skin at a very early age, along with xerosis, scaling, and telangiectasia. Speckled hypo- and hyperpigmentation and hyperkeratoses are also typical. These changes are well illustrated in Figs. 392 and 393. In early childhood, patients with xeroderma pigmentosum begin to develop cutaneous malignancies: basal cell and squamous cell carcinomas, and, less commonly, melanomas. The mortality from this disease is caused by destructive local growth of tumors and by metastases. In addition, patients may suffer from severe neurologic dysfunction, including mental retardation. Although no treatment is available, individuals with this disease benefit from a lifestyle which allows minimal exposure to sunlight.

12

Ichthyoses and Disorders of Keratinization

Figure 394

Figure 395

Ichthyosis vulgaris This is the mildest and most common form of ichthyosis, with an incidence in school-aged children as high as 1:250. It is inherited as an autosomal dominant trait and is present in a significant percentage of individuals with atopic dermatitis. It is not present at birth. The clinical appearance of this ichthyosis differs, depending on location. Figure 394 illustrates the fine, bran-like scaling on the upper chest. On the anterior lower leg, there are often larger, plate-

like scales which resemble the skin of a fish (Fig. 395). Facial involvement is usually minimal, and flexural areas are typically spared. Children with ichthyosis vulgaris are likely to have increased skin markings on the palms and soles and a high incidence of keratosis pilaris (see Figs. 252–254). Ichthyosis vulgaris tends to worsen in the wintertime when there is less sweating and lower humidity.

Figure 396

Figure 397

Ichthyosis vulgaris This figure illustrates the fine scaling of ichthyosis vulgaris and the conspicuous sparing of the flexures. Treatment of ichthyosis vulgaris centers around the use of emollients and creams and ointments containing urea and lactic acid. Excessive bathing and the use of alkaline soaps should be avoided. The exacerbation that frequently occurs in winter months can be lessened if a humidifier is used in the child's room.

Histopathology of ichthyosis vulgaris The histopathologic picture of ichthyosis vulgaris of autosomal dominant inheritance is diagnostic. In the illustration, one sees the stratum corneum to be dense and moderately hyperkeratotic, and the stratum malpighii to be essentially normal except for the absence of a stratum granulosum. This combination of hyperkeratosis (without parakeratosis) and absence of the granular layer is unique to this type of ichthyosis.

Figure 398

Figure 399

Bullous ichthyosis (epidermolytic hyperkeratosis) This condition is a rare, chronic, and often severe genodermatosis that is inherited in autosomal dominant fashion. The appearance of bullous ichthyosis in the newborn is illustrated in Fig. 398. Typically, there are large areas of denuded skin, and sometimes there are intact blisters. The differentiation from epidermolysis bullosa can usually be made by positive family history, the presence of subtle areas of hyperkeratosis, and, most important, the characteristic skin biopsy (see Fig. 403). Treatment in the newborn period should focus on gentle

handling to avoid new blister formation, the maintenance of fluid and electrolyte balance, and the prevention of bacterial superinfection. Over time, the generalized blistering resolves, and widespread areas of thick hyperkeratosis and scale develop. In Fig. 399 there is a mixed picture; focal erosions are present on the arms and abdomen, and there are areas of thick, discolored, furrowed hyperkeratosis. Note the predilection, which is not seen in ichthyosis vulgaris, for the antecubital fossae and intertriginous spaces.

Figure 400

Figure 401

Bullous ichthyosis (epidermolytic hyperkeratosis) These are further illustrations of the kind and severity of dyskeratinization that can occur in this condition. Figure 400 shows the process in typical areas: the palms, wrists, and knees. For some patients, severe involvement of the palms and soles creates a particular disability. Figure 401 shows bullous ichthyosis in its most severe and generalized form. Patients with this kind of extensive disease face a very difficult set of problems. Bacterial colonization of this thickened and furrowed skin may result in an extremely unpleasant body odor.

This foul smell, along with the disfigurement caused by the disease itself, may interfere enormously with social adaptation. Finally, some children remain prone to mechanically induced blisters in areas of friction or trauma. Antibacterial soaps are of some help in reducing odor. Treatment with keratolytics will often induce painful superficial erosions, and the use of oral retinoids, with all of their side effects, has met with little success. Fortunately, in many patients the disease tends to localize to smaller, usually flexural, areas with advancing age.

Figure 402

Figure 403

Bullous ichthyosis (epidermolytic hyperkeratosis) (cont.) Figure 402 shows a localized lesion in the popliteal space. Notice the degree of hyperkeratosis and the sculptured character of the skin markings. When there is only local involvement, the clinical picture can be indistinguishable from epidermal nevus. Patients with minimal involvement, like this, may have relatives with severe, generalized disease. Prenatal diagnosis by fetoscopy and fetal skin biopsy and by the recovery of epidermal cells in amniotic fluid is now possible. The exact nature of the defect in bullous ichthyosis is not known.

Histopathology of bullous ichthyosis The histopathologic pattern seen in bullous ichthyosis distinguishes it from the other ichthyoses. It is termed *epidermolytic hyperkeratosis*, or *granular degeneration*. A compact and hyperkeratotic stratum corneum overlies an abnormal upper spinous and granular cell layer. At this level there is a form of intracellular vacuolization and numerous clumped keratohyalin granules. Electron microscopy reveals excessive tonofilaments and keratohyaline granules.

Figure 404

Figure 405

Congenital ichthyosiform erythroderma This rare autosomal recessive condition may present with a collodion membrane at birth. The severity of the disease during infancy and later childhood is extremely variable. The most typical appearance features widespread scaling and moderate to severe erythroderma. The children with most severe involvement may experience difficulty with temperature regulation. Improvement sometimes occurs at puberty.

Erythrokeratoderma variabilis This is a rare autosomal dominant condition characterized by migratory areas of erythema and distinct plaques of hyperkeratosis. From an early beginning in infancy, there occur figurate and rapidly (within days) shifting areas of bright erythema on the face, anterior trunk, buttocks, and extensor aspects of the limbs. These may be brought on by changes in environmental temperature. In addition, there are fixed and localized hyperkeratotic plaques.

Figure 406

Figure 407

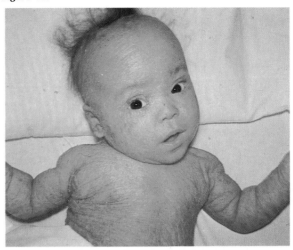

Lamellar ichthyosis *Collodion baby* is a descriptive term for the child who is born encased in a taut parchment-like membrane, accompanied by ectropion and eclabium. The outcome of this process is unpredictable. A small group of infants shed their membrane and develop completely normal skin; their condition is termed *lamellar exfoliation of the newborn*. Some go on to develop nonbullous congenital ichthyosiform erythroderma or Netherton's or Conradi's syndromes (see Figs. 414–417). Still others, like the infant in Fig. 406, have the chronic and severe autosomal recessive

disease lamellar ichthyosis. Collodion babies, irrespective of the cause, are very often born prematurely. In addition, they are at risk for cutaneous infection, sepsis, pneumonia, and hypernatremic dehydration and require careful supportive therapy. The infant in Fig. 407 was formerly a collodion baby and has gradually sloughed his membrane. At several months of age one can detect the beginnings of generalized hyperkeratosis and scaling. His underlying disease is lamellar ichthyosis.

Figure 408

Figure 409

Lamellar ichthyosis This figure shows in detail the kind of ichthyosis that gradually becomes established after the disappearance of the collodion membrane. Note the mosaic pattern of the scales and tendency of the edges of the scale to curl away from the surface. The scales are sometimes compared to armored plates. Bulla formation does not occur in this condition.

Lamellar ichthyosis Note that the entire skin surface, including the face, is affected by the hyperkeratotic, scaly, dyschromic dyskeratinization. Involvement tends to be most severe in flexural areas, as in the axilla pictured here. The metabolic defect in classic lamellar ichthyosis is unknown; some investigators consider this disease a dysfunction of epidermal differentiation. Topical therapy with the alpha-hydroxy acids, such as lactic acid, is somewhat helpful in reducing the amount of scale and improving appearance.

Figure 410

Figure 411

Lamellar ichthyosis (cont.)   The child in Fig. 410 has the severe degree of involvement that is an almost invariable feature of lamellar ichthyosis. Note the ectropion and tightness of the facial skin as a result of hyperkeratosis. The same compromised mobility of skin obtains on other parts of the body. Figure 411 illustrates involvement of the palms with thick hyperkeratosis and deep grooves. Not pictured here are the changes that may involve hair and nails. Scaliness of the scalp may be accompanied by partial hair loss. In addition, the nails may be ridged or thickened, and there may be thick subungual hyperkeratosis.

Figure 412

Figure 413

Histopathology of lamellar ichthyosis   In lamellar ichthyosis there is merely a variable degree of hyperkeratosis. The thickened stratum corneum is generally dense (and here shows an artificial separation from the subjacent stratum malpighii), and the stratum granulosum may be somewhat thickened, which is in marked contrast to its absence in ichthyosis vulgaris. The condition cannot be distinguished from the X-linked variety of ichthyosis by microscopy.

Palmoplantar keratoderma   There is a long list of genodermatoses that include thickening of the palms and soles as either the principle or an associated abnormality. The most common among all of these is Unna-Thost palmoplantar keratoderma. The autosomal dominant inheritance of this condition is illustrated by the mother-son involvement shown here. Treatment consists of the use of keratolytic agents to remove callus.

Figure 414

Figure 415

Netherton's syndrome This rare autosomal recessive syndrome manifests itself in a unique ichthyosis and hair shaft abnormality. The most distinctive cutaneous feature is termed *ichthyosis linearis circumflexa,* a collection of circinate, erythematous and hyperkeratotic lesions with a very characteristic double-edged scale along the margin. Alternatively, patients with Netherton's syndrome may have a generalized ichthyosiform erythroderma. The associated hair abnormality is seen in Fig. 414. Microscopic examination of these "bamboo hairs" most often reveals a hairshaft abnormality termed

trichorrhexis invaginata, a ball-and-socket insertion of the distal hair shaft into the proximal hair. There may also be pili torti (Fig. 767) or trichorrhexis nodosa (Fig. 765). The hair disorder tends to correct itself as time goes on. Patients with Netherton's syndrome tend to have an atopic diathesis, with some combination of asthma, allergic rhinitis, and eczematous dermatitis. The last of these is illustrated in Fig. 415. Finally, there is a tendency toward impaired cellular immunity and developmental delay.

Figure 416

Figure 417

Cutaneous manifestations of Conradi's disease Conradi's disease, or chondrodysplasia punctata, is actually a group of related syndromes that have differing prognoses and modes of inheritance. Skin changes are seen in some of the patients with each of the disease subtypes. The newborn may present as a collodion baby (see Fig. 406). In early infancy, there develops a generalized, whorled ichthyosiform erythroderma, as illustrated in these two photographs. Over time, the areas of ichthyosis are replaced by blotchy hyperpigmentation and

then, sometimes, by follicular atrophoderma. Patchy alopecia also may occur. Systemic features of chondrodysplasia punctata include stippling of the epiphyses, shortening of the femur and humerus, congenital cataracts, and saddle nose. The autosomal recessive form, also termed *rhizomelic dwarfism,* is most severe and usually causes psychomotor retardation and seizures. Those patients with the autosomal dominant disease (Conradi-Hunermann syndrome) have a generally better prognosis.

Figure 418

Figure 419

Cutaneous manifestations of Sjögren-Larsson syndrome   This is a rare autosomal recessive genodermatosis that is characterized by spasticity, mental retardation, and congenital ichthyosis. A combination of scaling and erythroderma is seen in the newborn. Over time, the ichthyosis tends to localize to the lower abdomen (Fig. 418) and flexural areas

(Fig. 419). There may be mild involvement of the palms and soles. The combination of spasticity and psychomotor developmental delay is often quite severe and may be accompanied by a seizure disorder. A specific retinal lesion, socalled glistening dots, is present in almost all patients with Sjögren-Larsson syndrome after 1 year of age.

Figure 420

Figure 421

Recessive X-linked ichthyosis   This disorder is characterized by ichthyosis that begins at or shortly after birth and persists through adult life. The "dirty" brown and tightly adherent scales are illustrated in both photographs. The scaling tends to favor the trunk and the extensor surfaces of the extremities. There is relative sparing of the face and flexural areas. The palms and soles are also spared, and the hair and teeth are normal. Most patients note marked improvement during the summer months, probably related to improved skin hydration.

Asymptomatic corneal opacities on the posterior membrane serve as an adult marker for this disease. In addition, there is a significant incidence of cryptorchidism in individuals with this syndrome. The locus for this rare genodermatosis is now known to be on the distal short arm of the X chromosome, and the disease is inherited in X-linked recessive fashion. The underlying metabolic disorder is a deficiency in the enzyme steroid sulfatase. Diagnosis can be confirmed by serum lipoprotein electrophoresis.

Figure 422

Figure 423

Linear epidermal nevus (systematized type) Widespread epidermal nevi sometimes occur. This condition was formerly termed *ichthyosis hystrix*. Patients with extensive lesions are especially prone to abnormalities in a variety of other organ systems—the epidermal nevus syndrome. Associated cutaneous lesions include hemangiomas, café-au-lait spots, and areas of hypopigmentation. Mental retardation and seizure disorder may also be present. Skeletal abnormalities seen in the epidermal nevus syndrome include limb hypertrophy, bone cysts, and incomplete formation of certain bones. A higher than normal incidence of malignancy, particularly Wilms' tumor, has also been associated with this disorder. All children with epidermal nevi should have a careful physical examination, and laboratory evaluation should be pursued as indicated.

Figure 424

Figure 425

Linear epidermal nevus This lesion consists of verrucous, hyperkeratotic papules which are closely grouped in a linear array. Epidermal nevi are often present at birth but may arise during the first year of life, and occasionally later. They may occur on the head and neck, trunk, or extremities. Lesions of the appearance illustrated in this figure are sometimes termed *nevus unius lateris*. Epidermal nevus has no malignant potential, except for the rare development of basal cell carcinoma in a preexisting lesion. Surgical treatment is required only when indicated for cosmetic considerations.

Inflammatory linear verrucous epidermal nevus (ILVEN) This linear array of pruritic papules arises most often during childhood. The lesions are erythematous and scaling and are usually localized to the lower extremities. At times, this entity may be difficult to distinguish from psoriasis. The persistence of inflammation in one anatomic area and the absence of psoriatic lesions elsewhere favor the diagnosis of ILVEN. Histologically, it may resemble psoriasis or nonspecific chronic dermatitis.

Figure 426

Figure 427

Acanthosis nigricans   This is a descriptive term for a velvety or varicose brown-to-black area of hyperkeratosis. The axilla is the most common location, but lesions are also seen on the posterior neck and in the groin. Less commonly, there is involvement in the antecubital and popliteal fossae, on the knuckles, and in other nonflexural areas. Onset may occur

during childhood or adult life. The histologic pattern is that of hyperkeratosis and papillomatosis; the brownish discoloration seems to be caused by these surface changes rather than by any local increase in the amount of melanin. Illustrated here are lesions of acanthosis nigricans on the anterior neck and in the axilla.

Figure 428

Figure 429

Acanthosis nigricans   Based on the varying etiologies, acanthosis nigricans is divided into several types. The title *benign acanthosis nigricans* is used to describe an autosomal dominant genodermatosis. The condition may develop at birth or during childhood and often intensifies after puberty. A second type, which heralds the presence of an associated malignancy (usually adenocarcinoma), is extremely rare during childhood. So-called *pseudoacanthosis nigricans* refers to the form that is directly related to obesity. It is not unusual to see this

condition on the nape of the neck or in the axilla and groin in an obese adolescent. This form of acanthosis nigricans frequently improves or resolves completely with dieting and weight loss. Finally, acanthosis nigricans may occur as a manifestation of several unrelated syndromes. These include Rud's syndrome, Bloom's syndrome, and Crouzon's syndrome. The relationship between acanthosis nigricans and insulin-resistant diabetes mellitus is discussed in the legend to Fig. 617.

Figure 430

Figure 431

KID syndrome The keratitis-ichthyosis-deafness (KID) syndrome is a multisystem disorder which in its most severe forms may be disabling. Cutaneous changes consist of thick keratoderma of the palms and soles, keratotic plaques on the face and extremities, and a diffuse ichthyosis with follicular accentuation. The presence of abnormal keratinization may be present at birth. Alopecia, nail dystrophy, and hypoplastic teeth are all part of this disorder. The hearing impairment in this disease is progressive and due to neurosensory deafness. Keratitis begins during childhood and is accompanied by neovascularization. Visual loss may be severe. Recurrent and atypical cutaneous infections may also be seen in KID syndrome.

Figure 432

Figure 433

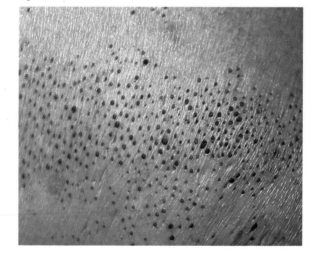

Acrokeratosis verruciformis This autosomal dominant disorder is characterized by numerous flat-topped or verrucous hyperkeratotic papules that are usually localized to the dorsae of the hands and feet. They tend to recur after surgical removal. Histologically, there are distinctive elevations of the epidermis that resemble church spires. It should be noted that patients with Darier's disease (see Figs. 308 and 309) may have identical acral lesions.

Nevus comedonicus The lesions in this condition consist of numerous clustered papules, each with a dark, central hyperkeratotic plug. The individual papules are clinically and histologically identical to the comedones seen in acne vulgaris. However, these nevoid plaques, which are often linear in configuration, do not necessarily occur in the ordinary sites of predilection of comedonal acne. Lesions may be single or multiple, and palm and sole involvement occurs. This may be a form of epidermal nevus.

13

Urticarial, Purpuric, and Vascular Reactions

Figure 434

Figure 435

Urticaria A *wheal* is an edematous papule that may enlarge to form a pink, sharply circumscribed elevated plaque. The typical lesions of urticaria, pictured here, have a suggestion of central clearing. By definition, the individual lesions of urticaria evolve quickly and resolve within 24–48 hours. They are usually accompanied by severe pruritus. The most common etiologies of urticaria are medications, foods, and viral and bacterial infections. Autoimmune disease and malignancy are extremely rare causes. In the child with chronic urticaria, it is often difficult or impossible to identify a single cause.

Cholinergic urticaria This type of urticaria is causally related to elevation in body temperature and sweating. The lesions usually develop rapidly after the beginning of exercise and resolve rapidly and spontaneously with cooling. The urticaria that develops in this condition has a typical appearance, illustrated here. The lesions consist of red or flesh-colored papules 2–3 mm in diameter that are surrounded by an ill-defined erythematous macule. The use of antihistamines will decrease the frequency and severity of attacks. Doxepin may also be effective.

Figure 436

Figure 437

Physical urticarias There are urticarias in which stroking, pressure, cold, heat, or sun exposure are causative. Figure 436 is whealing in linear form produced by stroking the skin with a degree of force that would ordinarily cause nothing more than transient erythema. The phenomenon, called *dermographism,* is present in a small percentage of normal individuals. Figure 437 is a huge wheal produced by resting an ice cube on the forearm. Cold-induced urticaria may be acquired or inherited. In the most common, acquired form,

patients develop lesions shortly after ingesting cold foods or liquids or shortly after exposure to a drop in environmental temperature. Patients with this form of sensitivity are at risk for laryngeal edema or circulatory collapse as a result of significant cold exposure. Antihistamines or doxepin are of some help in preventing attacks. In a very rare syndrome, contact of the skin with water, without respect to its temperature, produces wheals (aquagenic urticaria).

Figure 438

Figure 439

Erythema multiforme   This disorder is titled *multiforme* because the morphology of its lesions is so variable. The primary lesion is most often an erythematous macule that evolves into a papule. Early in the course, these lesions may easily be mistaken for urticaria. As the lesions enlarge, they form round or irregularly shaped plaques. The central area may blister or become dusky in color; this change represents the necrosis of keratinocytes in areas of active involvement. Concentric circles of erythema and dark gray discoloration

may evolve, forming the typical "target" lesion of erythema multiforme. The "target" lesions may coalesce and develop annular or serpiginous borders. Figure 438 is an overview of a severe case. In Fig. 439 there is a close-up of the target-like quality of the variably sized and shaped plaques. Note the redness and edema at the border and the duskier appearance at the center. Erythema multiforme tends to be acral in distribution, and the dorsum of the hand is a particularly common location.

Figure 440

Figure 441

Erythema multiforme   The type of bulla that may occur in erythema multiforme is shown here. Mucosal lesions are not uncommon. Erythema multiforme is a self-healing disease, with an average duration of about 2 weeks. Herpes simplex infection is by far the most common etiologic agent. Pulmonary infection with *Mycoplasma pneumoniae* is another well-documented cause of erythema multiforme in children and young adults. Finally, a wide variety of drugs, most commonly the sulfonamides, may cause this syndrome.

Histopathology of erythema multiforme   The term *erythema multiforme* is used differently by different authors, but all agree that an eruption that lasts only a few weeks and has iris (target) lesions is probably the disease in classic form. In the microscope, such lesions, prior to blister formation, generally show damage to the dermoepidermal junction with the formation of individual eosin-staining keratinocytes. The mild dermal inflammation is of mononuclear cells.

Figure 442

Figure 443

Erythema elevatum diutinum This is a rare skin disease which is characterized by purple or yellowish papules, nodules, and plaques that tend to cluster on the hands, feet, and extensor extremities. The skin overlying joints is a favored location. The distribution is usually symmetrical, and the disease tends to be chronic. Lesions of erythema elevatum diutinum may be asymptomatic but in some cases are painful. Figure 442 shows typical nodules and plaques on the elbow: yellowish papules on the finger are seen in Fig. 443. The etiology of this chronic leukocytoclastic vasculitis remains unknown, but an immune-complex etiology has been suggested. Dapsone is one mode of treatment.

Figure 444

Figure 445

Sweet's syndrome (acute febrile neutrophilic dermatosis) This syndrome is characterized by painful, raised, erythematous plaques and nodules. The cutaneous eruption is accompanied by spiking fevers and a neutrophilic leukocytosis. This condition is seen most commonly in middle-aged women, but it does occur in children. Skin biopsy reveals a widespread infiltrate of polymorphonuclear leukocytes throughout the dermis. Sweet's syndrome is often associated with either malignancy or antecedent infection. Systemic corticosteroids are the treatment of choice.

Erythema annulare centrifugum This is an erythematous and edematous lesion that gradually enlarges to form annular, polycyclic, and gyrate shapes. The lesions tend to resolve spontaneously but may reappear. Erythema annulare centrifugum has been attributed to a wide variety of causes. In some cases, it is temporally related to the development of malignancy and resolves with treatment or removal of the tumor. In other patients, the disease has been related to superficial fungal infections and a wide variety of viral and bacterial diseases.

Figure 446

Twin-to-twin "transfusion"   Twins who develop with some form of common circulation in utero may show a temporary difference of cutaneous color related to oddities of hemodynamics. In the picture one sees twin neonates of whom the one on the right is uniformly and abnormally erythematous, whereas the other is abnormally pallid. The one looks plethoric; the other, anemic. In the course of time, restoration of normal blood counts and color will develop in both.

Figure 447

Harlequin dyschromia   The word *harlequin* connotes, among other things, the quality of being parti-colored. The picture is of an infant in whom the left half of the trunk is pale and the right half red. The anomaly is transient and depends on circulatory derangement by gravity. If the child pictured were to be turned on its left side, which is now pale, that side would become red and the right side, now red, would become pale. This phenomenon is much more common among preterm infants.

Figure 448

Purpura   Hemorrhage into the skin takes many forms in structure, shape, and color. What we generally designate as purpura are macular lesions that may be punctate (petechial) or diffuse and red-purple in color (ecchymotic). The causes are numerous. Most common among the benign pigmented purpuras is Schamberg's disease, a disorder of unknown etiology. Affected children have numerous discrete patches of petechiae on the lower extremities. The individual lesions evolve into typical brown-orange macules containing "cay-

Figure 449

enne pepper'' spots. Fresh petechiae occur in other sites. More significant causes of purpura include septicemia (see Figs. 525–528), a wide variety of hematologic disorders, and vasculitis. Palpable purpura is, in fact, the hallmark of leukocytoclastic vasculitis. Leukocytoclastic vasculitis may be a manifestation of bacterial or viral infection, drug allergy, connective tissue disease, or cryoglobulinemia. Henoch-Schoenlein purpura, a common cause of childhood leukocytoclastic vasculitis, is discussed in Figs. 454–456.

Figure 450

Figure 451

Traumatic purpura The illustrations show hemorrhage into the skin occasioned by difficult passage of newborns through the birth canal. Such events are common, and as long as the hemorrhage is into skin alone, no great or lasting harm results. In Fig. 450 one sees edema and ecchymosis that resulted from molding of the head in a prolonged but spontaneous delivery. Figure 451 shows a hematoma of considerable size from a similar event. Modern obstetrics, which encompasses prenatal study of the maternal pelvis, radiography if necessary for that purpose and for unusual fetal size, sedation, muscle relaxants, anesthesia during delivery, and cesarean section when indicated, has tended to make serious traumatic purpura of these sorts less common. Nevertheless, in severe cases of traumatic hemorrhage of this kind, radiography for the possibility of skull fracture is good practice.

Figure 452

Figure 453

Traumatic purpura Throughout life hard knocks in the physical sense are the lot of all of us. Rupture of capillaries is exceedingly common in consequence, and more extensive rupture of arterioles, vesicles, arteries, or veins is common enough. Petechiae, ecchymoses, vibices, and hematomas are banal, nearly everyday events. The black eye and contusions are in everybody's experience. The illustration is a traumatic ecchymosis that may well represent a hickey ("passion purpura").

Purpura fulminans This condition is a rare and exceedingly serious consequence of certain acute infectious diseases. Scarlet fever of bygone days, meningococcal meningitis, severe varicella, and congenital protein C deficiency have been known to be complicated by fulminating purpura that went on to gangrene, extreme toxicity, shock, and death. The cause of the condition seems to be necrotizing vasculitis attended by defects of clotting (disseminated intravascular coagulation).

Figure 454

Figure 455

Henoch-Schoenlein purpura Palpable purpura is but one aspect of a syndrome that is marked also by attacks of arthralgia, abdominal pain, and hematuria. The entire complex of visible cutaneous purpura, arthralgia, and visceral signs and symptoms results from a widespread vasculitis. In addition to purpura, as shown in Fig. 454 on the buttocks and in Fig. 455 around an ankle, the skin may show edematous plaques, vesicles, and even necroses. Without the cutaneous signs, arthralgia might mislead one to consider rheumatic fever; abdominal pain might suggest an acute surgical abdomen and lead to unnecessary laparotomy; and hematuria might mislead to diagnoses like glomerulonephritis or nephrolithiasis. Good clinical judgment, however, will confirm the diagnosis of Henoch-Schoenlein purpura. The cause of this condition is not known. The prognosis is usually good, except for the rare child who goes on to develop chronic nephritis.

Figure 456

Figure 457

Henoch-Schoenlein purpura This picture is a good representation of both the purpuric elements and the edema that may appear in the Henoch-Schoenlein syndrome. In itself, without signs and symptoms of hemorrhagic consequences or edema in joints, gut, or kidneys, many another diagnosis would have to be differentially considered in an appearance like this.

Idiopathic thrombocytopenic purpura This autoimmune condition is triggered by causes unknown and is manifest by intracutaneous bleeding. The purpura takes the form of petechiae and ecchymoses not only in the skin, where it is obvious, but also in the oropharyngeal mucous membranes and in the nose and gastrointestinal tract. The illustration is of ecchymosis in the pinna of an ear.

Figure 458

Aphthous stomatitis This very common condition is characterized by recurrent episodes of painful ulceration on the lip, tongue, or buccal surfaces. The individual lesions quickly evolve from erythematous macules to papules, and then to yellowish ulcerations with a surrounding pink or red halo. The etiology is not known, and the ulcers heal in 7 to 10 days without scarring. Whereas a solitary lesion is the cause of only temporary, minor discomfort, there are some individuals who develop deeper and larger ulcers, or numerous erosions. For them, aphthous stomatitis can be a severe problem.

Figure 459

Behçet's syndrome This rare disease is characterized by a classic triad of recurrent ulcerations of the oral mucosa, genital ulcers, and eye involvement. The oral ulcers, one of which is pictured here, tend to be larger, more numerous, and more frequently recurrent than those of simple aphthous stomatitis. Genital lesions occur on the penis and scrotum in males, and on the vulva in females. These frequently recurrent ulcers tend to heal with scarring. The various forms of eye involvement include uveitis and keratoconjunctivitis and may eventuate in blindness.

Figure 460

Behçet's syndrome The sharply marginated oral ulcers of this syndrome are pictured in Fig. 460. Figure 461 shows the typical genital lesions. Other cutaneous lesions may be widespread and include papules, vesicles, abscesses, and lesions of erythema nodosum. In addition to the eyes and skin, a number of other organ systems may become involved. Severe chronic arthritis and thrombophlebitis are common occurrences. Gastrointestinal disease ranges from mild ab-

Figure 461

dominal discomfort to chronic diarrhea and an ulcerative colitis-like illness. Neurologic manifestations, including recurrent meningoencephalitis and brain stem lesions, are often the most serious and can be life threatening. Diagnosis of Behçet's syndrome is based on the presence of the typical clinical findings. The disease is difficult to treat, but immunosuppressive drugs and corticosteroids are the most frequently used therapies.

14

Bullous, Pustular, and Ulcerating Diseases

Figure 462

Figure 463

Pemphigus vulgaris   Pemphigus vulgaris is a rare autoimmune bullous disease which occasionally occurs during childhood. The disease affects both the skin and mucous membranes and can be life threatening. The typical lesions of pemphigus vulgaris are pictured here. Erosions of the lips, gums, tongue and palate, as pictured in Fig. 462, are a common presenting symptom and may be misdiagnosed early in the course of the disease. The difficulty in chewing and swallowing that

may occur can become a significant complication. Cutaneous lesions consist of flaccid weeping blisters which quickly erode to leave large denuded areas of skin. Nikolsky's sign, the extension of blistering by lateral finger pressure, is seen in the presence of widespread disease. Figure 463 shows the kind of crusting that develops as the roofs of blisters of pemphigus vulgaris disintegrate.

Figure 464

Figure 465

Pemphigus vulgaris   The blisters of pemphigus vulgaris may arise on an erythematous base, or on normal-appearing skin, as pictured here. A variety of modalities have been employed in the treatment of this disease. The patient who is seriously ill requires hospitalization. For most, the most rapid and effective treatment remains high-dose systemic steroids. Patients undergoing this form of therapy are at high risk for infection and must be followed with extreme care. Other useful therapies are immunosuppressive agents, such as azathioprine, gold, and plasmapheresis.

Histopathology of pemphigus vulgaris   Biopsy of a lesion of pemphigus vulgaris reveals a blister within the epidermis, the base of which is one or two cells above the basal layer. The underlying pathologic process is the loss of cohesion between epidermal cells, termed *acantholysis*. There is relatively little inflammatory infiltrate; acantholytic cells can be seen within the blister cavity. Direct immunofluorescence shows IgG and complement in the intercellular spaces of the epidermis. Indirect immunofluorescence is also positive for a specific intercellular substance-reactive antibody.

Figure 466

Pemphigus vegetans When the cutaneous changes of pemphigus take place in intertriginous spaces, clear blistering is not evident. Rather, one sees boggy inflammation and tumid granulation. The essential histologic process is again epidermal acantholysis, but blister roofs part almost at once and secondary infection is inevitable. The figure is a good representation of the kind of clinical appearance that develops in pemphigus vegetans. Lesions on other parts of the body take the form of pemphigus vulgaris.

Figure 467

Pemphigus foliaceus This figure illustrates the type of scaling that accompanies pemphigus foliaceus. What one sees is largely exfoliating stratum corneum, not blisters. On biopsy, there is acantholysis occurring high in the epidermis, usually in the granular layer. There may be a subcorneal cleft, but the rest of the epidermis remains attached. The autoantibodies which are seen by immunofluorescence are identical to those in pemphigus vulgaris.

Figure 468

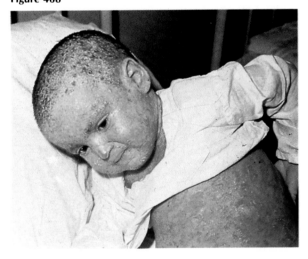

Pemphigus foliaceus This form of pemphigus is less severe than pemphigus vulgaris because blister formation occurs higher in the epidermis. As a result, there is less compromise of vital cutaneous functions. In most areas of the world, pemphigus foliaceus is extremely unusual in children. In Brazil, there is an endemic form of pemphigus foliaceus, termed *fogo selvagem,* which affects individuals of all ages. Pictured here are the typical lesions of pemphigus foliaceus.

Figure 469

The disease often begins in the scalp with areas of erythema and scaling. As it progresses to involve the trunk and extremities, there evolve numerous crusting and erythematous plaques. Severe scaling is common, but there is usually no blister formation and no involvement of the oral cavity. Treatment consists of topical or systemic steroids, depending on the severity of the disease.

Figure 470

Figure 471

Pemphigus erythematosus This is the least serious form of the pemphigus group of diseases and is probably best considered as a localized form of pemphigus foliaceus. It is unusual in children but does occasionally occur. Typically, there is scaling and crusting in a ''butterfly distribution'' on the face, and also involvement of the chest, back, and scalp. The disease may be mistaken for severe seborrheic dermatitis or systemic lupus erythematosus. Biopsy of a lesion of pemphigus erythematosus reveals an intraepidermal bulla in the upper layers of the epidermis. As in all forms of pemphigus, IgG antibody to intercellular substance is present in the serum. Pemphigus erythematosus tends not to be a severe disease; most cases can be controlled with topical steroids alone.

Figure 472

Figure 473

Subcorneal pustulosis (Sneddon-Wilkinson disease) This condition is most common during adulthood, but it does occur in children. Characteristically, crops of vesicles and pustules (Fig. 472) spring up and evolve into areas of superficial crusts and scales. As the lesions coalesce, they form the type of arcuate plaque that is illustrated in Fig. 473. The most common locations are the axillae, groins, and flexures of the upper and lower extremities. The lesions are often pruritic, and, especially in childhood, there may be fever and an elevated white blood count. The etiology of this condition is completely unknown. Diagnosis is best confirmed by classic histologic appearance, which consists of collections of neutrophils just beneath the stratum corneum. The disease process is essentially benign, but dapsone is an effective therapy for the patient with frequent or severe recurrences.

Figure 474

Familial benign chronic pemphigus (Hailey-Hailey disease)
This blistering disease is inherited in autosomal dominant
fashion. Onset tends to occur during late adolescence. Patients
with this disorder have a pruritic vesicular eruption in
intertriginous areas that is worse during the summer months.
Intact bullae may be absent and there is often only an erosive
and crusted intertrigo in the axillae, groins, and on the neck.
Control of this condition is best achieved by the avoidance
of the causative factors, such as heat or friction, and the
treatment of superinfection when it occurs.

Figure 475

Epidermolysis bullosa simplex   This autosomal dominant condition is among the mildest of the diseases that are termed
epidermolysis bullosa. The exact deficit is not known but is
postulated to be an abnormal structural protein or a cytolytic
enzyme. Epidermolysis bullosa simplex begins at birth or in
early infancy, and throughout life the site of blistering
corresponds to areas of friction or other trauma. During
infancy, blisters occur on the neck, lower extremities, and
hands and feet. In the child who is old enough to wear shoes,
the dorsal toes are a common site of bulla formation.

Figure 476

Epidermolysis bullosa simplex   In this condition, cleavage
occurs through the basal cell layer of the epidermis, and the
dermoepidermal junction is otherwise undisturbed. The result
is that the lesions are superficial in appearance, and cutaneous
function is well preserved. Very importantly, the lesions of
epidermolysis bullosa simplex heal without scarring. In children with this disorder, mucous membrane involvement is
minimal, and usually does not produce serious difficulty.
There may be some nail dystrophy, but this also heals with
the cutaneous process.

Figure 477

**Recurrent epidermolysis bullosa of the hands and feet (Weber-
Cockayne type)**   This particular variant of epidermolysis
bullosa involves only the hands and feet; the cleavage plane
is above the basal layer. The lesions tend to first appear
during late childhood and adolescence. Pictured here are
blisters on and near the great toe; the appearance of the
bullae is modified by the thickness of the stratum corneum
in this area. Patients with this disease tend also to suffer
from hyperhidrosis. Minimizing trauma to the hands and feet
and the use of antiperspirants help prevent blister formation.

Figure 478

Figure 479

Epidermolysis bullosa dystrophica The autosomal recessive, dystrophic form of epidermolysis bullosa is a multisystem disease which is characterized by chronic and recurrent subepidermal blistering. The disorder often leads to severe disability, interfering with the normal processes of growth and development. Blister formation usually begins at or shortly after birth, and intraoral involvement may lead to early feeding difficulties. Normal handling of the infant with this disease results in the formation of tense bullae, which quickly evolve into ulcerations. The typical blisters, crusts,

and erosions of dystrophic epidermolysis bullosa are seen in Fig. 478. The most serious sequelae of this disorder are due to the fact that the blisters heal with scarring. The recurrent episodes of bulla formation and healing on the hands and feet may result in an acquired syndactyly, as illustrated in Fig. 479. In the esophagus, the same process eventuates in mechanical obstruction. The strictures that form lead to nutritional difficulties, and even perforation or squamous cell carcinoma of the esophagus. Eye involvement, with ulcers, keratitis, and opacities, is an additional problem.

Figure 480

Figure 481

Epidermolysis bullosa dystrophica This figure shows a foot with complete destruction of the toenails, induced syndactyly of the fourth and fifth toes, and typical wrinkled scarring of the skin surface. Appropriate care for the child with epidermolysis bullosa must begin in the nursery and involves the use of topical dressings to protect eroded skin and the careful handling of the infant to avoid new blister formation. Subsequent management includes efforts to minimize skin trauma, good dental and ophthalmic care, and careful attention to diet and nutrition.

Epidermolysis bullosa (albopapuloid of Pasini) This is a dystrophic form of epidermolysis bullosa which is inherited in autosomal dominant fashion. Widespread blistering may be present at birth. During puberty, patients with this disorder develop distinctive ivory-white follicular papules on the chest and lower back. The albopapuloid form of epidermolysis bullosa has been associated with a defect in anchoring fibrils. The prognosis tends to be good.

Figure 482

Epidermolysis bullosa dystrophica (dominant) This figure illustrates another patient with a dominant form of scarring epidermolysis bullosa. The Cockayne-Touraine form tends to begin during infancy and is associated with widespread blistering and milia formation. Shown here are a number of tense bullae on the flexor surface of the arm. Mouth involvement and nail dystrophy may also occur.

Figure 483

Epidermolysis bullosa atrophicans gravis This disorder, also known as *epidermolysis bullosa letalis,* is a severe variant. The bullae are junctional, and the disease is inherited in autosomal recessive fashion. Extensive cutaneous involvement is often present from birth. Severe erosions of the oral mucous membrane are commonplace and lead to early feeding difficulties. Gastrointestinal involvement leads to severe dysphagia, pyloric stenosis, or chronic malabsorption. Lesions in the genitourinary and respiratory systems are additional problems. Most patients do not survive into adulthood.

Figure 484

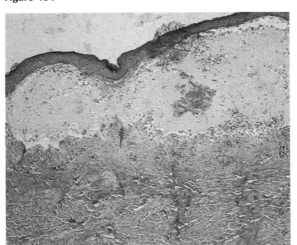

Histopathology of epidermolysis bullosa Random biopsy of a vesicle of epidermolysis bullosa is generally of no help in distinguishing types of the disease. All show the nonspecific picture of a subepidermal blister. A biopsy taken from a newly formed, preferably induced, vesicle is helpful if the subepidermal basement membrane is stained with PAS. Then the bulla may be seen formed through the basal cells, just above or just beneath the basement membrane. Electron microscopy is of particular value in establishing an exact diagnosis.

Figure 485

Figure 486

Chronic bullous dermatosis of childhood This is a distinct blistering disease which occurs exclusively during childhood, most commonly during the first 5 years of life. The disorder is characterized by large, tense bullae which tend to occur in the genital area, lower abdomen and back, and lower extremities. The degree of pruritus is variable. Figure 485 illustrates the particular fashion in which the blisters tend to

cluster. Note the circular or oval configuration of blisters. As an early lesion heals with crusting and hyperpigmentation, new lesions arise in a string of pearls or rosette-like pattern along the periphery. The blisters themselves may be elongated or sausage-shaped. Figure 486 shows the clustering of tense blisters on the inner thighs. This is probably the most common location for chronic bullous dermatosis of childhood.

Figure 487

Figure 488

Chronic bullous dermatosis of childhood These two figures show the annular and polycyclic clustering of blisters that is so typical of this disorder. Biopsy of a lesion reveals a subepidermal blister with an infiltrate of neutrophils and/or eosinophils. Immunofluorescence is more distinctive and usually shows a linear deposit of IgA along the basement membrane (in the lamina lucida). In most patients, there are also circulating IgA antibodies directed against the basement membrane. For most affected children this is a self-limited

disease, and it resolves spontaneously over a period of several years. Sulfapyridine and dapsone are the most effective therapies. These drugs have hemolytic activity, and the patients must be monitored for induced anemia and methemoglobinemia. A test for adequate glucose-6-phosphate dehydrogenase should be done before initiation of therapy, and hemoglobin determinations should be made subsequently until stabilization occurs.

Figure 489

Figure 490

Dermatitis herpetiformis This intensely pruritic papulovesicular eruption is fairly unusual during childhood. Figure 489 shows the symmetrical distribution of the grouped, excoriated lesions on the extensor extremities and buttocks. Additional papules and vesicles on the upper chest and face are seen in Fig. 490. Dermatitis herpetiformis is a disease that affects both the skin and gastrointestinal tract. The majority of children with this disorder have a gluten-sensitive enteropathy. This may lead to diarrhea and malabsorption, or it may

be evidenced only by villous atrophy on jejunal biopsy. The approaches to treatment of this disease include sulfapyridine or dapsone and a gluten-free diet. As mentioned above, children treated with dapsone or sulfapyridine must be carefully monitored for the development of hemolytic anemia. Adherence to a diet which contains no gluten is extremely difficult but, if accomplished, will often lead to prolonged remission.

Figure 491

Figure 492

Dermatitis herpetiformis This picture of lesions of dermatitis herpetiformis shows them in a highly characteristic distribution on the back. Because of the intense pruritus, excoriations tend to outnumber the primary papulovesicles. Direct immunofluorescence of perilesional skin is an effective means of confirming the diagnosis of dermatitis herpetiformis. Typically, there are granular deposits of IgA at the tips of the dermal papillae.

Histopathology of dermatitis herpetiformis Biopsy of erythematous and edematous skin around a blister is helpful in establishing the diagnosis of dermatitis herpetiformis. Such a specimen tends to show the unique histologic features, namely, the formation of neutrophilic microabscesses in papillary bodies. The individual papillae show crescentic empty spaces between the epidermis and the cellular infiltrate.

15

Cutaneous Manifestations of Systemic Disease

Figure 493

Figure 494

Cutaneous expressions of systemic lupus erythematosus Figure 493 illustrates cutaneous involvement of systemic lupus erythematosus (SLE) in the classic butterfly pattern on the face. This macular and intensely erythematous eruption is frequently aggravated by sun exposure and may flare with other symptoms of systemic disease. Figure 494 shows the temporary alopecia which is also a hallmark of SLE. This

autoimmune disease of unknown etiology affects almost every organ system. The most common findings in the child with SLE are fever, arthralgias, and arthritis. In addition, pleuritis, pericarditis, and central nervous system involvement are frequently seen in children with SLE. Lupus nephritis develops in the vast majority of affected children and may eventually cause renal failure.

Figure 495

Figure 496

Cutaneous expressions of systemic lupus erythematosus These photographs illustrate additional cutaneous features of SLE. The lesions on the back (Fig. 495) and the hands (Fig. 496) are intensely erythematous macules and slightly edematous papules and plaques. Childhood SLE occurs most frequently during adolescence and is more common among blacks and among girls. The diagnosis is established by meeting four of eleven clinical and laboratory criteria. Clinical criteria include

rash (either malar or discoid), photosensitivity, oral ulcers, and disease of the joints, lungs, kidney, and central nervous system. The single most reliable laboratory test is antinuclear antibody, which will be positive in almost every case of childhood SLE. Other laboratory criteria include leukopenia, thrombocytopenia, and the presence of anti-native DNA antibodies. Adrenocorticosteroids remain the mainstay of therapy for SLE.

Figure 497

Figure 498

Neonatal lupus erythematosus This condition is probably due to the transplacental passage of anti-Ro (SSA) antibodies from mother to infant. The mother may suffer from a form of connective tissue disease or may be completely asymptomatic. The infants pictured in Figs. 497 and 498 were born with these atrophic and telangiectatic plaques on the face. The lesions may also resemble those of subacute cutaneous lupus in the older patient. The skin lesions, which are more

common in girls, tend to resolve without scarring. Nonfluorinated topical steroids and avoidance of the sun are the only treatments that may be required. A frequent complication of neonatal lupus is congenital heart block. This situation is potentially life threatening and may sometimes require implantation of a pacemaker. Although neonatal lupus is self-limited, there are reports of affected infants going on to develop connective tissue disease during adolescence.

Figure 499

Figure 500

Discoid lupus erythematosus Illustrated here is the characteristic plaque of a discoid lesion of lupus erythematosus. There is a violaceous hue at the border and central atrophy with scarring. Similar involvement in the scalp can cause permanent alopecia. Discoid lesions may be a cutaneous manifestation of systemic lupus erythematosus or the sole physical finding in a disease that does not go on to affect any other organ system. Treatment consists of avoidance of the sun or the use of sunscreens, antimalarial agents, and topical or intralesional corticosteroids.

Histopathology of lupus erythematosus The diagnosis of discoid lupus erythematosus is based on clinical and histologic morphology. The histologic features are keratotic follicular plugs, vascular dilatation beneath the epidermis, damage to the dermoepidermal interface, patchy collections of lymphocytes, and loss of pilosebaceous units.

Figure 501

Figure 502

Dermatomyositis This collagen vascular disease is characterized by a combination of symmetrical proximal upper and lower extremity muscle weakness and cutaneous disease. Early symptoms of muscle involvement include general malaise, difficulty in playing or climbing stairs, myalgias, and muscle tenderness. These illustrations are highly characteristic of the cutaneous part of the syndrome. Figure 501 shows symmetrical, intense, erythema and edema of the face. The violaceous color of the periorbital rash is sometimes described as heliotrope in hue; the edema is so intense that it makes

the face look puffy. Erythematous and edematous papules and plaques may also be present on the dorsum of the hand (Fig. 502), and on the elbows and knees. The lesions which occur over the distal interphalangeal joints are referred to as Gottron's papules. An additional cutaneous finding, which is particularly characteristic of childhood dermatomyositis, is calcinosis cutis. This may present as firm, superficial nodules or plaques or as painful deposits of calcium in muscle or fascia.

Figure 503

Figure 504

Dermatomyositis These illustrations show more of the cutaneous manifestations of dermatomyositis. Figure 503 again shows the classic Gottron's papules, and in Fig. 504 there is a nearly identical process on and around the elbow. In both these pictures, the cutaneous disease has advanced to wrinkling and atrophy. The diagnosis of dermatomyositis is usually made on the basis of elevated muscle enzymes (especially creatinine phosphokinase and aldolase), electromyography,

and muscle biopsy. Skin biopsy tends not to be helpful in differentiating dermatomyositis from other collagen vascular disease. Early therapy with systemic corticosteroids is vital in the treatment of both muscular and cutaneous disease and in the prevention of calcinosis. In contrast to the adult form of the disease, childhood dermatomyositis is not associated with malignancy.

Figure 505

Figure 506

Scleroderma (progressive systemic sclerosis) This is a multisystem connective tissue disease that is relatively rare in childhood. Patients may suffer from arthritis and muscle weakness, and from the results of pulmonary, esophageal, cardiac, and renal involvement. The condition of the skin on the face and hands is shown in Fig. 505. The induration and hidebound quality are hard to capture in photography, but they can be imagined from the fixed expression in the face

and from the exposure of the teeth by the indurated lips, and on the hands from the pallor of the knuckles and seeming inflexibility of the fingers. If the patients were undressed, the chest would likely be judged to be hidebound, too, from the outline of the ribs and its general shape. Figure 506 shows scleroderma on a leg and a foot, the latter also scarred from ulceration. Again photography cannot bring out the hardness of the skin as palpation can.

Figure 507

Figure 508

Scleroderma (progressive systemic sclerosis) This figure of fingertips shows the pallor of Raynaud's phenomenon and telangiectasia. The patient also has scleroderma of the hands, forearms, and face. If calcinosis cutis were present or supervened, this type of case would be designated as the CRST syndrome, i.e., marked by calcinosis. Raynaud's phenomenon, sclerodactyly, and telangiectasia. Such a combination is the most severe of the cutaneous possibilities of progressive systemic sclerosis.

Histopathology of scleroderma The biopsy specimen, oriented here with the surface to the left, shows nothing abnormal in the epidermis or dermis. The essential changes are in the subcutis on the right and consist of increased cellularity and replacement of fat cells by newly formed, abnormal connective tissue. Fibrosis and sclerosis of the underlying fascia may also be present.

Figure 509

Figure 510

Cutaneous expressions of rheumatic fever and rheumatoid arthritis Erythema marginatum is a specific cutaneous expression of rheumatic fever. An unusually good representation of erythema marginatum at a static moment is shown in Fig. 509. As the title says, the condition is redness in the form of margination. What is not told is that the red margination is about normal-appearing skin and that it is transient and recurrent over days and weeks, and may precede cardiac or joint symptoms or signs. Rheumatoid arthritis sometimes has a cutaneous expression that is of the nature of urticarial dermographism or edematous erythema provoked by scratching, especially during a febrile period of the illness. An illustration of it is Fig. 510. Persistent and transient stripes of erythema and edema are shown on the back and buttocks.

Figure 511

Figure 512

Cutaneous expressions of polyarteritis nodosa This multisystem disease is a form of necrotizing vasculitis that affects small and medium-sized arteries. Frequent areas of systemic involvement are the gastrointestinal tract and kidneys. Palpable purpura are the most common cutaneous manifestation of this disease. In addition, there may be necrotic ulcers and distal gangrene. Tender cutaneous nodules are occasionally seen, but these are more characteristic of benign cutaneous periarteritis nodosa, which has no systemic manifestations.

Cutaneous expressions of chronic granulomatous disease This X-linked recessive inherited disorder is characterized by recurrent granulomatous infections of multiple organ systems. The underlying defect is in the neutrophils' inability to produce hydrogen peroxide and to kill bacteria; this abnormality can be verified by the nitroblue tetrazolium slide test. Pneumonia, meningitis, and septicemia are among the most serious complications of this disease. An intertriginal eczematous eruption and granulomatous nodules and plaques are among the cutaneous manifestations.

Figure 513

Figure 514

Sarcoidosis This is a disease of unknown etiology which is characterized by the formation of noncaseating granulomas in many different organ systems. Sarcoidosis is more common among blacks. It is unusual in children, but it does occur. During childhood, the most common presenting signs and symptoms are lymphadenopathy, uveitis, and cutaneous disease. In very young children, arthritis, eye disease, and skin

disease tend to predominate. Children with sarcoidosis may also have weight loss, fever, and respiratory involvement. Disorders of calcium metabolism are evidenced by hypercalcemia and hypercalcuria. Figures 513 and 514 illustrate the erythematous and flesh-colored papules that may be the sole cutaneous manifestation of sarcoidosis. Systemic steroids remain the treatment of choice in this disease.

Figure 515

Figure 516

Sarcoidosis Here illustrated are highly characteristic papules of sarcoidosis on and around the eyelids. Similar lesions are common around the nose and mouth. Sarcoidosis such as this may be cutaneous only, or, more likely, may involve other organs. Investigation for systemic disease should include x-rays of the lungs and pulmonary function tests. The eyes should be examined for uveitis and lacrimal gland enlargement.

Histopathology of sarcoidosis Sarcoidosis, whatever may be its single or multitudinous causes, shows a consistently uniform histologic picture. That picture in skin or any other organ is a "naked" tubercle consisting of epithelioid and giant cells with few or no lymphocytes and no necrosis. These collections or granulomas in the skin may be small or large, discrete or confluent, and situated superficially or deeply in the dermis. In the photomicrograph, so-called naked tubercles are seen superficially placed.

Figure 517

Cutaneous manifestations of Crohn's disease This chronic inflammatory bowel disease has several cutaneous manifestations. Most common are perianal fissures, fistulas, and granulomatous nodules. The exophytic lesions pictured here could easily be confused with condylomata acuminata. Metastatic Crohn's disease may present with ulcerations in intertriginous folds. Children with Crohn's disease may also suffer from erythema nodosum and aphthous ulcers.

Figure 518

Cutaneous manifestations of thalassemia major The homozygous form of thalassemia (thalassemia major, Cooley's anemia) presents with a severe hemolytic anemia during infancy or early childhood. Affected children are usually small for their age and have distinctive frontal bossing, along with jaundice and hepatosplenomegaly. Illustrated here are the chronic leg ulcers that are fairly common in this hematologic disorder.

Figure 519

Cutaneous manifestations of sickle cell anemia Leg ulcers, commonly around the malleoli, are a frequent manifestation of sickle cell anemia. In size, shape, and appearance they are very similar to stasis ulcers. The occurrence of leg ulcers in sickle cell anemia is attributed to sludging of the sickled cells, local ischemia, and stasis. Treatment consists of bed rest, occlusive or semi-occlusive dressings, and the use of topical and oral antibiotics when superinfection is present. Oral zinc therapy may be of value.

Figure 520

Pyoderma gangrenosum This form of gradually enlarging necrotic ulceration usually involves the distal lower extremity. Typical characteristics include a purulent base and a purplish, undermined border. Etiologies include inflammatory bowel disease, chronic active hepatitis, and Behçet's syndrome. Arthritis may be an associated finding. Treatment consists of bed rest, local care, and the injection of intralesional steroids along the border of the lesion. Dapsone, sulfapyridine, and oral corticosteroids are additional therapies.

Figure 521

Figure 522

Kawasaki's disease This childhood disease of unknown etiology is officially diagnosed by the presence of high fever lasting 5 or more days, and 4 of the following criteria: conjunctival injection, mucous membrane changes, rash, erythema or edema of the palms and soles, and cervical lymphadenopathy. A common cutaneous finding during the second week of illness is desquamation of the palms and soles, and, very frequently, the perineum. Systemic aspects of Kawasaki's disease include arthritis, aseptic meningitis, and hydrops of the gallbladder. Coronary artery aneurysms develop in 20 percent of patients who are not treated, and some children go on to develop myocardial infarction. Current therapy, consisting of aspirin and intravenous gammaglobulin, seems to reduce the incidence of cardiac disease. Children who do not meet the strict diagnostic criteria for Kawasaki's disease should be treated as if they did, if there is a strong clinical suspicion. All children with Kawasaki's disease should be followed with serial two-dimensional echocardiography.

Figure 523

Figure 524

Necrobiosis lipoidica This condition has some resemblance to granuloma annulare, more resemblance histopathologically than clinically, but the two conditions are far from being the same. For one thing, the lesions of necrobiosis lipoidica are generally much larger than those of granuloma annulare. (The lesions in Fig. 523 are exceptional, probably because the disease is in early development; Figure 524 is more typical for size.) The border is not ringed with papules, and the center, unlike in granuloma annulare, is eventually atrophied or scarred. Ulceration may occur. Necrobiosis lipoidica does not improve spontaneously or with reasonable treatment to the point of *restitutio ad integrum* as granuloma annulare does. The condition is common in diabetes mellitus wherewith it is distinguished by addition of the term *diabeticorum*. Frequently it is seen in patients who themselves do not have diabetes, but often those patients have familial histories of consanguineous relatives with diabetes mellitus.

Figure 525

Figure 526

Cutaneous effects of *Pseudomonas* sepsis   Sepsis caused by *Pseudomonas aeruginosa* occurs most commonly in the child with an underlying illness. It is seen in children with immune deficiency due to cancer chemotherapy, in those with malnutrition, and in those with extensive burns. Some of the less specific cutaneous manifestations, specifically erythematous macules and petechiae, are pictured in Figs. 525 and 526. *Pseudomonas* sepsis may also present with small, discrete nodules and bullae. The classic skin lesion of *Pseudo-*

monas sepsis is termed *ecthyma gangrenosum*. This form characteristically progresses quickly from a well-circumscribed area of edema, to a centrally located blister, to a gangrenous ulcer with a gray eschar. Multiple lesions in different stages of evolution may be present, and the lesions may appear on any body surface. Gram stain and culture of tissue scraped from the base of a blister will be positive for *Pseudomonas*.

Figure 527

Figure 528

Cutaneous effects of meningococcemia   The early treatment of meningococcemia with appropriate parenteral antibiotics can often be lifesaving. Cutaneous manifestations of this disease may provide the single most important diagnostic clue in the acutely ill child. The most common finding on the skin are petechiae and purpura. The small petechial lesion pictured in Fig. 527 develops early in the course of the disease, and a scraping yields gram-negative diplococci on both Gram stain and culture. Subsequently, the lesions arise

in additional crops, enlarge in size, and coalesce. The numerous ecchymoses pictured in Fig. 528 are the result of this rapidly ongoing process. These areas may become necrotic and develop eschars. Other cutaneous manifestations, occurring subsequently, include peripheral gangrene and purpura fulminans, with confluent areas of necrosis of the skin. These are the result of vasospasm, shock, and a consumption coagulopathy. A deficiency in protein C may play a particular role in this process.

Figure 529

Figure 530

Cutaneous effects of gonococcemia Infection with *Neisseria gonorrhoeae* may manifest as a purulent conjunctivitis in the newborn or as a genital discharge in the sexually abused child or sexually active adolescent. Disseminated gonococcal infection, as illustrated here, is quite rare. Gonococcemia presents with a migratory polyarthralgia or septic arthritis, and fever. The skin lesions are few in number, are often located on extremities, and may overlie the involved joints. Initially, there are small erythematous macules that progress to papules. These tender lesions may develop a small vesicle and then a gray, umbilicated center. Rarely, bullae, petechiae, and larger hemorrhagic lesions are also seen. The two photographs show the macules and necrotic papules that are typical of disseminated gonococcal infection.

Figure 531

Cutaneous effects of endocarditis (Janeway lesions) Mucocutaneous lesions are common in subacute bacterial endocarditis. The erythematous and hemorrhagic macules shown here are termed *Janeway lesions*. They may occur on the distal finger pads, palms, or soles. Other manifestations of this disease include petechiae on the oral mucosa and skin and splinter hemorrhage under the nails. Large, painful nodules or areas of gangrene involving the fingers or toes are signs of embolus formation.

Figure 532

Figure 533

"Leiner's disease" The infant pictured here has a severe generalized erythroderma with diffuse scaling. A similar condition was described by Leiner, a Viennese dermatologist, at the turn of the century. Over subsequent years, the term "Leiner's disease" has been used to describe children with severe and widespread seborrheic dermatitis, diarrhea, failure to thrive, and recurrent infections. Certain cases of this clinical syndrome seemed to have been associated with a specific dysfunction of the fifth component of complement. Although the nosologic position of Leiner's disease remains controversial, it is most likely that this clinical presentation (erythroderma, diarrhea, and growth failure) may result from a variety of immunologic abnormalities. A complete evaluation of the immune system in an infant like the one pictured here is mandatory.

16

Cutaneous Manifestations of HIV Infection

Figure 534

Cutaneous manifestations of HIV infection (chronic varicella zoster infection)   This figure illustrates a form of infection with varicella zoster virus that is unique to patients with immune suppression from HIV. The 6-year-old child pictured here developed recurrent vesicular and ulcerative lesions of the trunk and extremities following an episode of chickenpox. The lesions contain numerous multinucleated giant cells and are culture-positive for varicella zoster virus. This form of infection responds to treatment with intravenous acyclovir but tends to recur when therapy is discontinued.

Figure 535

Cutaneous manifestations of HIV infection (scarring from herpes zoster)   This 3-year-old girl developed herpes zoster as an early manifestation of her immune deficiency. Despite therapy with intravenous acyclovir, severe scarring resulted. Herpes zoster occurs more frequently in children who have had chickenpox very early in life. Although herpes zoster is certainly seen in the healthy child, its occurrence in a child who is at risk for HIV infection should signal concern.

Figure 536

Cutaneous manifestations of HIV infection (candidal parony-chiae and nail dystrophy)   Candidiasis is the most common mucocutaneous manifestation of pediatric HIV infection. Children with AIDS or lesser forms of HIV-related disease frequently develop oral thrush, which recurs or persists despite topical antifungal therapy. Recalcitrant infections of the diaper area and neck folds are also common. Illustrated here are chronic paronychiae with a resultant nail dystrophy.

Figure 537

Cutaneous manifestations of HIV infection (drug eruption)   Drug eruptions, usually due to therapy with trimethoprim-sulfamethoxazole, are particularly common among children with HIV infection. This young girl developed a rash subsequent to treatment with that drug for *Pneumocystis carinii* pneumonia. Biopsy of the skin lesion illustrated here revealed an interface dermatitis. A generalized blanchable erythema and true Stevens-Johnson syndrome may also be seen. The frequency of drug eruptions in children with AIDS illustrates the complex effect of HIV on the immune system.

Figure 538

Cutaneous manifestations of HIV infection (chronic herpetic gingivostomatitis)   Children with AIDS frequently suffer from persistent herpetic infections of the mucous membranes or skin. The gingivostomatitis shown here would be typical of primary infection in a healthy child. One would then expect recurrences to be considerably milder. By contrast, the child with HIV infection may have recurrent episodes of gingivostomatitis or may develop infection which does not respond at all to acyclovir.

Figure 539

Cutaneous manifestations of HIV infection (seborrheic dermatitis)   Seborrheic dermatitis occurs with particular severity in individuals who are infected with HIV. The infantile form consists of severe scaling and erythema of the scalp, flexural areas, and, sometimes, the entire skin surface. The last resembles the clinical appearance of the child with so-called Leiner's disease. Illustrated here is an older child with recalcitrant inflammation in the skin folds behind the ears. She also had severe crusting and scaling of the entire scalp.

Figure 540

Cutaneous manifestations of HIV infection (leukocytoclastic vasculitis)   Occasionally, chronic leukocytoclastic vasculitis occurs in children who are infected with HIV. It is not certain whether this is the direct result of this virus or of some other concurrent infection. The palpable purpura seen here on the lower extremities are indistinguishable from those observed in Henoch-Schoenlein purpura. The chronicity of this patient's eruption, however, was atypical, and pointed to the possibility of HIV-related disease.

Figure 541

Cutaneous manifestations of HIV infection (condylomata acuminata)   Children who are infected with the human immunodeficiency virus are prone to a wide variety of viral infections. Lesions caused by human papillomavirus may be unusually widespread and persistent. A case of condylomata acuminata in a one-year-old girl is illustrated here. Extensive flat warts or periungual warts may also be seen.

17

Disorders of the Dermis (Infiltrates, Atrophies, and Nodules)

Figures 542

Circumscribed scleroderma (morphea)   There are conditions that take the title scleroderma but are not related to progressive systemic sclerosis. They are marked by areas of hardened skin, small or large, scattered or localized, single or multiple, and of variable shape. Here illustrated is localized or circumscribed scleroderma in the form of several discrete lesions of different shapes, all confined to the skin of the left side of the chest. The lesions are firm and atrophic.

Figure 543

Circumscribed scleroderma (linear, en bande)   Illustrated is a type of circumscribed scleroderma that is linear in shape and situated on the flexor aspect of a leg, extending from the medial aspect of the thigh through the popliteal space to near the Achilles tendon. Again the affected skin is hard, slightly depressed, and dyschromic. Extensive areas of linear morphea are the most difficult to treat. There is a tendency toward permanent deformity, in the form of atrophy or contractures.

Figures 544

Circumscribed scleroderma (en coup de sabre)   Here is another kind of hardened skin in the form of a depression, as though the result of a blow from a blunt instrument or a weapon like a saber. Location on one side of the brow is highly characteristic. Such lesions are seen with no other associated anomaly or as part of hemiatrophies. Atrophy or absence of subcutaneous fat is also part of such a process.

Figure 545

Circumscribed scleroderma (morphea)   This kind of circumscribed scleroderma is highly characteristic. The solitary or individual lesion of the condition is a circle or oval of firm skin that is whitish, slightly depressed, and surrounded by a different color that is lilac or purple. There may be but one such lesion of moderate size or many of about the same size or very large ones covering large areas of skin. The course of the condition is variable, too. Spontaneous recovery in children is common.

Figure 546

Circumscribed scleroderma (morphea)   Illustrated here is a lesion of morphea resolving. From an appearance like that in Fig. 545, the lesion has become reddish, has risen to the level of the surrounding skin, and will eventually leave nearly completely or with minor dyschromia. The cause of circumscribed scleroderma of any form is unknown.

Figure 547

Atrophoderma (Pasini-Pierini)   This condition is most common in adolescent girls, and the etiology is completely unknown. Characteristically, there develop single or multiple well-circumscribed, slightly hyperpigmented areas of cutaneous atrophy, with a sharp "cliff-drop" border. The lesions tend to enlarge slowly, and then persist. Some believe that this form of atrophoderma represents a variant of morphea, in which atrophy is more evident than is sclerosis.

Figure 548

Histopathology of atrophoderma (Pasini-Pierini)   Atrophy of the skin may involve epidermis, its appendages, dermal collagen and elastic tissue, adipose tissue, or combinations thereof. In atrophoderma of Pasini and Pierini, the atrophic process is limited strictly to the dermal collagen. The two specimens shown here represent markedly atrophic skin on the right and comparable uninvolved skin from the same patient on the left.

Figure 549

Histopathology of lichen sclerosus et atrophicus   The most constant histologic feature of this condition, well illustrated here, is a zone directly beneath the epithelium that is sparse of cells, pale, and almost "sclerotic." Separating this abnormal zone from the deeper, uninvolved corium is a horizontal, patchy band of mononuclear inflammatory cells. The epithelium may show hyperkeratosis, atrophy, and liquefaction degeneration of the stratum malpighii, features that do not appear in this photomicrograph.

Figure 550

Figure 551

Lichen sclerosus et atrophicus (cont.) These two figures illustrate lichen sclerosus et atrophicus in its most typical location. This cutaneous disorder is more common in girls and is usually confined to the skin surrounding the anogenital region. The onset of the disease may be accompanied by pruritus, burning, or vaginal discharge, or it may be completely asymptomatic. Porcelain-colored or slightly erythe-

matous macules gradually coalesce to form plaques. The end result is an area of induration and shiny atrophy in an hourglass shape around the rectum and vagina. Childhood lichen sclerosus et atrophicus tends to be a self-limited disease, with improvement occurring at the time of puberty. The use of topical corticosteroids provides some symptomatic relief and may hasten the resolution of the process.

Figure 552

Figure 553

Lichen sclerosus et atrophicus In Fig. 552, discrete and confluent ivory-colored macules are shown on an area of skin that might be of the trunk, arms, or thighs. Extragenital lesions tend to be asymptomatic. Figure 553 illustrates lichen sclerosus et atrophicus involving the ankle, which is not an

unusual location. Another common site is the male genitalia, especially the foreskin and glans penis. The result may be a nonretractable foreskin, or stenosis of the urethral meatus. It appears that lichen sclerosus et atrophicus may be a common cause of phimosis in young boys.

Figure 554

Figure 555

Anetoderma (macular atrophy) The term *anetoderma*, meaning slack skin, is most often used to describe a form of cutaneous atrophy which has no clear preceding cause. Anetoderma is divided into two clinical types. The Jadassohn form of anetoderma, most common among girls, is characterized by the eruption of round, slightly erythematous macules over large areas of the trunk and proximal extrem-

ities. The lesions quickly evolve into small areas of atrophy, each with an outpouching of shiny white skin (Fig. 554). The second form of anetoderma bears the eponym Schweninger-Buzzi. This form, illustrated in Fig. 555, is distinguished by the slow evolution of lesions which arise without preceding inflammation.

Figure 556

Figure 557

Anetoderma (macular atrophy)   Here is another illustration of idiopathic macular atrophy. In this patient the lesions arose with no evidence of prior inflammation. Occasionally, skin changes that are similar to the primary anetodermas can be seen as a sequela of sarcoidosis, granuloma annulare, Hansen's disease, secondary syphilis, or penicillamine therapy. In either situation, the biopsy shows the localized loss of elastic tissue.

Histopathology of anetoderma   Anetoderma (macular atrophy), whether primary or secondary to some other dermatosis, shows a stereotypic histopathologic picture. The atrophy affects dermal elastica, and a special elastic tissue stain is required for its demonstration. The destruction of elastic tissue usually involves a spherical or ellipsoidal mass. In the photomicrograph, elastic tissue is absent in the right lower half of the field and is present adjacent to it.

Figure 558

Figure 559

Striae distensae Ruptures within the dermis in the lines of cleavage of the skin that are not associated with obvious external trauma are common in pregnancy and obesity. In pregnancy, mechanical stretching of the skin by the developing fetus and its housing and, in obesity, extreme storage of fat can be taken to be cause enough for dermal ruptures; but a factor of endocrinopathy or idiopathic response to hormone balance also seems to be operative. Athletes,

particularly weight lifters, sometimes show striae distensae, and again mechanical stretching and idiopathic hormonal influence may be adduced in explanation since the phenomenon is not universal. In Fig. 558 one sees striae on a back that may well be of a weight lifter; Figure 559 shows striae and telangiectasia in a patient who is and has long been on topical adrenocorticosteroids for good reason. The hormonal influence in the latter case is indubitable.

Figure 560

Figure 561

Connective tissue nevus This group of hamartomas may be composed of the various elements of the extracellular connective tissue: collagen, elastic fibers, or glycosaminoglycans. One example of the collagen variety is the shagreen patch, a cutaneous manifestation of tuberous sclerosis. These yellow or orange plaques of coalescent papules are often seen in the lumbosacral area. Other varieties of connective tissue nevus

are not associated with tuberous sclerosis. Particularly, collagenomas may be seen in solitary, eruptive, and multiple forms. The last of these is a familial disorder. Elastic fibers are found in isolated elastomas and in the small yellowish papules of the autosomal dominant Buschke-Ollendorf syndrome. The latter is also characterized by asymptomatic sclerotic densities of the bones.

Figure 562

Figure 563

Granuloma annulare   This benign condition is characterized by one or more circular plaques, consisting of rings of papules around a depressed center. Figure 562 is most typical; Fig. 563 is somewhat variant. The hands and feet are the commonest sites for the lesions of granuloma annulare. One or two lesions are the usual number. Occasionally, eruptive and widespread lesions are seen. For the most part, granuloma annulare is not associated with any other disease, nor is there any known cause. The condition is symptomless. It has been known to vanish spontaneously after a procedure such as a biopsy of part of it. Topical or intralesional corticosteroids are a standard therapy. Parent and child should be warned that the lesions may persist for months or years before response to therapy or spontaneous resolution. Recurrence may also occur.

Figure 564

Figure 565

Subcutaneous granuloma annulare (pseudo-rheumatoid nodule)   There is a form of granuloma annulare which presents with deep nodules. A more typical annular lesion may overlie the nodule or may be present at another anatomic site. These lesions are most frequently localized to the digits, scalp, dorsum of the feet, or anterior tibial region.

Histopathology of granuloma annulare   Granuloma annulare is a granuloma of a group that includes necrobiosis lipoidica and the nodule of rheumatoid arthritis and rheumatic fever. All have similar histopathologic pictures that cannot always be distinguished from one another without clinical correlation. Here, in a typical example of granuloma annulare, one sees a central zone sparse of cells, surrounded by mononuclear and multinucleated cells in palisade pattern.

Figure 566

Figure 567

Juvenile xanthogranuloma This is a common and completely benign cutaneous nodule. Typically, a juvenile xanthogranuloma is firm and dome-shaped. The lesion is reddish in color at first, as in Fig. 566, but develops a fairly typical orange-brown hue over time (Fig. 567). Most juvenile xanthogranulomas are located on the head or neck, as pictured in these two infants, but the lesions sometimes occur on the trunk or extremities. They may be present at birth, but most develop during the first year of life. Juvenile xanthogranuloma is not associated with abnormalities in serum cholesterol or triglyc-

erides, and the individual lesions undergo spontaneous involution, usually over a period of 1 to 2 years. A diagnostic biopsy is sometimes needed, but surgical intervention beyond this is certainly not required. A juvenile xanthogranuloma on the skin may be accompanied by intraocular lesions. For this reason, the physician must pay careful attention to the examination of the eyes. An abnormality in the color of the iris or an enlargement of the globe should trigger a prompt ophthalmologic referral.

Figure 568

Figure 569

Juvenile xanthogranuloma This photograph shows four lesions. It is somewhat more common to see multiple juvenile xanthogranulomas than a solitary lesion. Rarely, they may number in the hundreds. As mentioned, xanthogranuloma of the eye is the most common complication of this generally benign and self-limited condition. Multiple small juvenile xanthogranulomas seem to be slightly more common in children with neurofibromatosis, and these patients have an additional tendency toward juvenile chronic myelocytic leukemia.

Histopathology of juvenile xanthogranuloma This lesion, also designated *nevoxanthoendothelioma,* is a benign, localized histiocytoma. Because lipid is often present in such lesions, they qualify histologically as xanthomas. In addition to mononuclear, lipid-filled histiocytes, one finds multinucleated giant cells of a distinctive type (Touton) which have a ring of nuclei set in cytoplasm that is foamy at the periphery only. Touton giant cells are almost never seen in the xanthomas of systemic dyslipidoses.

Figure 570

Figure 571

Dermatofibroma These are benign dermal nodules which represent a focal proliferation of fibroblasts; the overlying epidermis is slightly thickened. Their occurrence is not unusual in children and adolescents. Dermatofibromas are firm and may be black, red, brown, or flesh colored. Their diameter generally ranges from 0.5 to 1.5 cm, although they may occasionally be larger. Dermatofibromas may be solitary or multiple, and they develop either spontaneously or after

minor trauma to the skin, such as an insect bite. Most are asymptomatic. A very useful diagnostic maneuver is executed by exerting lateral pressure on the lesion. The skin overlying a dermatofibroma will frequently dimple. Dermatofibromas require surgical treatment only when they are of cosmetic concern to the patient. However, biopsy is occasionally required in order to confirm the diagnosis and to differentiate it from more serious disorders.

Figure 572

Figure 573

Granular cell tumor These are unusual nodular lesions that vary from 0.5 to 3.0 cm in diameter. They may be single or multiple and are firm, elevated, and circumscribed. The tongue is a common site. The lesion pictured here is fairly typical of the cutaneous variety. The original name *granular cell myoblastoma* derived from an early theory that these tumors arise from immature striated muscle cells. In fact, Schwann cells are a more likely origin. The condition is benign and lends itself to any form of extirpation.

Benign cephalic histiocytosis This very distinctive eruption consists of numerous brownish-yellow macules and papules involving the head and neck. The mucous membranes are spared. Benign cephalic histiocytosis usually begins during the first 3 years of life, and the lesions continue to evolve for several years. The condition then resolves spontaneously during childhood but may leave small atrophic or pigmented scars. These children do not develop systemic disease and are not at risk for histiocytosis X. Electron microscopy of the histiocytic infiltrate reveals comma-shaped bodies in the cytoplasm.

Figure 574

Figure 575

Keloids The lesions pictured here are typical of the disfiguring changes that sometimes occur after trauma to the skin. In children, a laceration, surgical procedure, or a bout of chicken pox may be the inciting event for keloid formation. Figure 574 shows a keloid that was caused by ear-piercing. Keloid formation is more common in black than in white children, is very rare in infants, and becomes somewhat more frequent with increasing age. Keloids begin as firm, telangiectatic plaques confined to the site of the initial wound. Over time, they become less erythematous and extend beyond

the site of injury. Pruritus, burning, and hyperesthesia are frequent complaints. In contrast to hypertrophic scars, keloids do not resolve spontaneously. In fact, they may continue to grow over a period of years. The monthly injection of intralesional corticosteroids is currently the preferred treatment for most keloids. This modality is most successful in the newly forming keloid, which is softer and smaller than the well-established one. Surgical excision will almost always result in recurrence, but is somewhat more successful when accompanied by the injection of corticosteroids.

Figure 576

Figure 577

Keloids The keloid pictured here is a common variety that develops after a thermal burn. The irregular contour and crab-like projections are characteristic and illustrate the root of the word *keloid*: from the Greek word *chele*, meaning crab's claw. The size and thickness of lesions of this type make treatment difficult. The chest and back are also common sites for keloids of another cause, namely, inflammatory acne. In that situation, repeated injections of intralesional corticosteroids are often of cosmetic benefit.

Histopathology of keloids In many instances it is impossible clinically to distinguish a keloid from a hypertrophic scar. Distinction can, however, almost always be made histologically. Both lesions show proliferation of fibroblasts and collagen, but in keloids one finds in addition broad bands of hyalinized collagen separated by pale-staining areas. This particular histopathologic pattern is not seen in hypertrophic scars. Keloids, unlike hypertrophic scars, persist indefinitely.

Figure 578

Figure 579

Digital fibrous tumor of childhood   This is a rare fibromatosis that starts in infants as either a single or, less commonly, as several nodules. Parents may be alarmed by the rapid growth of the lesions. Digital fibrous tumors usually occur on the dorsal and sometimes on the lateral aspects of the distal phalanges of fingers and toes. They may be globular, red, and smooth as illustrated in Fig. 578, or reddish-brown and convoluted, especially when they wrap around digits, as

illustrated in Fig. 579. Deformity of the adjacent nail plate may occur. The lesions are benign and have never been known to become malignant and metastasize. Recurrence is a common event after surgical excision, but many such tumors will involute without treatment over a period of several years. In most cases, the best treatment is simple observation.

Figure 580

Histopathology of digital fibrous tumor of childhood   Fibro-matoses are localized overgrowths of mature fibrocellular and collagenous connective tissue. Dupuytren's contracture, Pey-ronie's disease, and the desmoid tumor of the rectus sheath are examples. Such processes have the ability to invade contiguous structures. Infantile digital fibromatosis is unique in that the fibroblasts contain round intracytoplasmic bodies, here distinctively stained red, the presence of which permits precise diagnosis.

Figure 581

Figure 582

Mastocytosis This is a set of disorders which are character-ized by the accumulation of mast cells in the skin and, sometimes, in other organs. There is a wide clinical variety. The plaque shown in Fig. 581 represents a solitary masto-cytoma, which occurs almost exclusively during infancy. This is most often a reddish-brown or orange nodule or plaque which is rubbery in consistency. There is occasionally a history of repeated blister formation on the surface. Figure 582 shows the numerous macules and papules of reddish or

brownish hue that are typical of *urticaria pigmentosa*. This generalized form is the most common type of mastocytosis, and it also usually develops during early childhood. The whealing of lesions when they are rubbed (Darier's sign) is virtually pathognomonic for this disorder. Mechanical trauma is thought to degranulate mast cells and cause a local release of histamine. Dermographism in uninvolved skin is not uncommon.

Figure 583

Figure 584

Mastocytosis Figure 583 is another good representation of the typical lesions of the skin, this time involving papules in great abundance and of red-brown hue. Figure 584 shows the same process in a black infant who, incidentally, has a large Mongolian spot on the lower part of the back above the buttocks. Patients who develop urticaria pigmentosa during early childhood tend to have only cutaneous involvement,

and their disease will almost always involute over a period of years. No treatment is necessary, but it is important to provide the parents with a list of medications that might cause the sudden and potentially life-threatening release of hista-mine. These include aspirin, codeine, morphine, polymyxin B, aminoglycosides, and nonsteroidal anti-inflammatories. Immersion in a very hot bath may have the same effect.

Figure 585

Figure 586

Mastocytosis Figure 585 illustrates the blister formation that may occur in infants with urticaria pigmentosa. Mast cells may sometimes be detected by staining the material from a scraped blister with Giemsa stain and examining it microscopically. Occasionally, a biopsy is necessary in order to differentiate bullous mastocytosis from other blistering diseases of infancy. Figure 586 is a photograph of the same patient in later life; he has gone on to develop diffuse infiltrative mastocytosis of the entire skin surface. The prog-

nosis in this rare form of the disease, and in individuals who first develop mastocytosis later in life, is not as good. Particularly common is involvement of the gastrointestinal and skeletal systems with the infiltrative process. Elevated urinary histamines or histamine metabolites are indicative of such widespread disease. Patients with this type of systemic mastocytosis are prone to attacks of pruritus, flushing, and hypotension. The massive release of mast cell products is sometimes fatal.

Figure 587

Figure 588

Histopathology of mastocytosis Mastocytosis most often involves the skin, producing the clinical picture known as urticaria pigmentosa. Histologic confirmation of the diagnosis depends on the demonstration of an excessive number of mast cells within the dermis. The biopsy should not be taken from a lesion that has been rubbed, because rubbing causes degranulation of the cells. In the lesions of children with the condition, mast cells are generally present in large numbers,

but when they are only slightly increased in number, a special stain is necessary to establish the diagnosis with certainty. In Fig. 587, one sees sheets of uniform mononuclear cells beneath the epidermis that are suggestive of the diagnosis. By use of a metachromatic stain, which specifically colors the heparin-containing cytoplasmic granules a violet or reddish color and other structures blue (Fig. 588), the diagnosis is confirmable.

Figure 589

Figure 590

Nevus lipomatosus superficialis Fat tissue is no more exempt from nevoid anomaly than is any other tissue. Here illustrated is a condition in which fat tissue is redundant and situated high in the dermis, well above its normal position in the hypoderm. The result is papillomatosis of yellowish hue and variable shape. There are no great consequences from the condition beyond the cosmetic, which may be remedied by plastic surgery in cases like the one pictured.

Leiomyoma There are several neoplasms of the skin that are notably tender or painful. Leiomyoma is of this class. The intense pain associated with it takes the form of unprovoked paroxysms that reach a crescendo of torture before subsidence. The lesions are fleshy papules or nodules of no great morphologic distinctiveness. They have no malignant potential. Surgical ablation is curative and simple enough for solitary lesions but may be more complicated for numerous and widely spaced lesions such as those illustrated.

18

Drug Eruptions

Figure 591

Figure 592

Drug eruptions (dermatitis medicamentosa) Drug eruptions have become common experiences to practitioners in all branches of modern medicine. The profusion of drugs now available, the continuous influx of new drugs, and the capability of drugs to cause actions different from or in addition to their pharmacologically desirable actions make adverse cutaneous reactions inevitable facts of modern medical practice. The kinds of cutaneous reactions are varied. Exanthems

(erythematous, morbilliform, or maculopapular), urticaria, fixed drug eruptions, and erythema multiforme are the most common. Both illustrations are of the morbilliform type of reaction: Figure 591 resulted from novobiocin and Fig. 592 from ampicillin. Constitutional symptoms of low-grade fever and malaise may be associated with such drug eruptions. Morbilliform eruptions from ampicillin are more frequently seen in children with infectious mononucleosis.

Figure 593

Figure 594

Drug eruptions (dermatitis medicamentosa) Drug eruptions may mimic nearly the entire range of dermatoses of other causes. One of the commonest forms is the exanthematic, the lesions of which are usually erythematous and edematous. Common causes of drug eruptions include ampicillin, cephalosporins, semi-synthetic penicillins, and barbiturates. We have just illustrated cases that were morbilliform. Illustrated here are cases clinically resembling erythema multiforme:

Fig. 593 resulted from a sulfonamide and Fig. 594 from a chloroquine (Plaquenil). Note again the tendency to universality and symmetry. Drug eruptions of the types so far illustrated may be uncomfortably pruritic and attended at their onset by prodromal malaise, but they are rarely serious and usually subside fairly quickly upon elimination of the causative drug and, on occasion, even in the face of continued administration of an absolutely required drug.

Figure 595

Figure 596

Fixed drug eruption Another common type of adverse reaction to drugs is the so-called fixed drug eruption. The term *fixed* is intended to suggest that the cutaneous change, occurring for the first time in given sites (anywhere), recurs in those same sites upon subsequent and repeated administration. Upon subsequent provocation, new reactions in new sites may occur, but original sites always flare again. There are several drugs that are well known for their propensity to cause fixed drug eruptions, namely, phenolphthalein, salicylates, phenacetin, barbiturates, antipyrine, arsenicals, and gold salts. The clinical morphology of a fixed drug eruption is usually a roundish plaque that is palpably edematous and purplish in color. Sometimes fixed drug eruptions are bullous. Both illustrations are of fixed drug eruptions caused by phenolphthalein.

Figures 597

Figure 598

Fixed drug eruption This cutaneous change appeared after institution of treatment of an unrelated condition with an antihistamine. The proof of a drug as cause of an eruption is sometimes certain on the basis of repeated experience, but often conjectural or circumstantial, especially in the case of newly introduced drugs. Proof by withdrawing a suspected drug and observing subsidence of the eruption and then reappearance upon resumption of the drug is usually not wise or safe practice.

Histopathology of fixed drug eruption Fixed drug eruptions are acute inflammatory plaques that tend to leave post-inflammatory hyperpigmentation upon resolution and to recur in the same sites upon readministration of the causative drug. During the inflammatory stage, the histopathologic changes are similar to those of erythema multiforme (Fig. 441). The changes are damage to the lower level of the epidermis and appearance of eosinophilic prickle cells and a mononuclear infiltrate. Often, there is melanin within macrophages in the upper dermis.

Figure 599

Figure 600

Toxic epidermal necrolysis (Stevens-Johnson syndrome) This is a severe generalized form of erythema multiforme which is almost always the result of a reaction to a medication. The most common agents are sulfonamides, anticonvulsants, and nonsteroidal anti-inflammatory drugs. Combinations of target lesions, bullae, and erosions are seen; the bullae occur especially on or around the lips, in the mouth, and on other mucous surfaces. Frozen section processing of a biopsy of toxic epidermal necrolysis allows for rapid diagnosis. In

patients with erosions and blisters, one sees necrotic keratinocytes, severe degeneration of the basal layer, and a subepidermal separation. The mortality rate in this disease is significant; most deaths are related to superinfection and sepsis. Patients with toxic epidermal necrolysis benefit enormously from intensive medical care, in a burn unit when possible. The role of systemic steroids in this disease remains extremely controversial.

Figure 601

Figure 602

Acute exanthem syndrome The anticonvulsant medications phenytoin (Dilantin), phenobarbital, and carbamazepine (Tegretol) each may cause this severe form of drug reaction. The mucocutaneous manifestations are strawberry tongue and a generalized scarlatiniform eruption which is followed by desquamation. The rash may also be purpuric. The presence of high fever, lymphadenopathy and hepatosplenomegaly may give the false impression of an infectious disease. Elevations in blood urea nitrogen, liver enzymes, and peripheral eosinophil count may also be present.

Gingival hyperplasia from phenytoin The mechanisms of adverse reactions to drugs vary. Some, like the urticarial or eczematous, are clearly based on an allergic or immunologic mechanism; others are utterly obscure in mechanism. Such is the gingival hyperplasia caused by phenytoin. Since it occurs in almost all patients receiving the drug, all one can say is that the effect probably is within the normal pharmacologic action of the drug.

Figure 603

Figure 604

Iododerma and bromoderma   Iodides and bromides are drugs that can cause severe adverse cutaneous reactions, and of these, the worst are acneform, furuncular, carbuncular, chancriform, pyodermatous, or granulomatous. Iodides and bromides are widely distributed, not only in foods and in the environment but also in proprietary and formally prescribed medicaments. The pictures are of still relatively minor consequences of adverse reactions from the two halides, of which bromides are usually worse than iodides. Lesions like those of acne or folliculitis caused by an iodide are shown in Fig. 603. Figure 604 is a granulomatous reaction caused by a bromide. Another baleful characteristic of drug eruptions from halides is persistence and extension of reaction once it occurs. The reason for such persistence or extension, even when a known source of the offending drug is removed, is the wide dispersion of occult iodine or bromine salts in foods, in the environment, and indeed in body-own chemistry. Iodine, for example, is a constituent of thyroid hormone.

Figure 605

Histopathology of bromoderma   The halides (bromine and iodine salts) may, in certain individuals, induce a variable combination of acute inflammatory and hyperplastic changes in the epidermis, which clinically may range from pustules to large, destructive, chancriform lesions. In the illustration, one sees surface crust, pseudocarcinomatous hyperplasia of the epidermis, and intense inflammation, mainly in the superficial dermis and subcutaneous fat. Eosinophils are often numerous in the cellular infiltrate.

19

Panniculopathies

Figure 606

Figure 607

Subcutaneous fat necrosis of the newborn This is a self-resolving and benign condition that is seen in healthy newborns. The infants develop single or multiple firm, red-purple nodules or plaques which are asymptomatic. Cheeks, back, buttocks, and thighs are the most common locations. Lesions may be present at birth, or they may develop during the first month of life. Most lesions resolve spontaneously over a period of 2–4 weeks, but some last significantly longer. There is usually no residual atrophy or scarring. It is difficult to capture the quality of panniculitis in photography, but a sense of it can be appreciated on the buttock of the patient pictured in Fig. 606. The etiology of this disorder is probably ischemic injury to subcutaneous fat. Lesions often develop at sites of pressure. Subcutaneous fat necrosis is occasionally associated with hypercalcemia.

Figure 608

Figure 609

Sclerema neonatorum Unlike the condition just described, sclerema neonatorum presents itself as symmetrical areas of induration on cheeks, shoulders, buttocks, and calves. The skin over involved subcutaneous fat is uniformly board-like, cold, and livid in color, as though frozen. Infants so affected appear rigid because mobility is interfered with by the sclerema, and they are severely ill. Mortality is high. The condition is more common in premature infants and in those with severe underlying disease, such as sepsis or dehydration.

Histopathology of subcutaneous fat necrosis of the newborn In this clinically dramatic, but essentially benign, condition, needle-shaped triglyceride crystals form and incite a foreign-body reaction characterized by giant cells. In tissue routinely processed, as here, the lipid has been dissolved by solvents, but one can still see thin protoplasmic strands that had separated the acicular crystals. Upon resolution, normal structure reappears.

Figure 610

Figure 611

Erythema nodosum Red, tender, subcutaneous nodules on the extensor aspects of the legs between knees and ankles are a common condition of many causes, some clear, some likely, and many obscure. The more important conditions that are heralded or attended by erythema nodosum are such infections as streptococcal upper respiratory infections, ul-cerative colitis, histoplasmosis, coccidioidomycosis, tuber-culosis, syphilis, and leprosy. Another condition which is sometimes revealed by investigation of erythema nodosum is sarcoidosis. Drugs appear to be the cause of particular cases of erythema nodosum. In many cases, however, no clear cause can be found.

Figure 612

Figure 613

Histopathology of erythema nodosum Erythema nodosum is a panniculitis. The panniculitides in general are difficult to distinguish clinically and microscopically, but of them, ery-thema nodosum is easiest to so distinguish. The inflammatory process affects chiefly the fibrous septa; the fat lobules are less involved. Here one sees pronounced inflammation of a septum diagonally cut and some involvement of the adjacent fat lobules. Scattered multinucleated giant cells are present.

Relapsing, febrile, nodular, nonsuppurative panniculitis (Weber-Christian) The panniculitis that is associated with the eponym Weber-Christian is well described by the adjec-tives in the above title. The condition recurs unpredictably (relapsing), is attended by fever (febrile), has lumpy lesions (nodular), and does not go to purulence (nonsuppurative).

Figure 614

Panniculitis from cold   Local exposure to cold leads to the formation of ice crystals within cells. Injury to cell contents occurs during both cooling and thawing. Cold panniculitis may occur in a child whose glove or boot has filled with snow. It is also seen in the youngster who has been sucking on a frozen dessert product—so-called popsicle panniculitis. The self-limited injury sustained in that condition is illustrated in Fig. 614.

Figure 615

Lipoatrophy (lipodystrophy)   The localized lipoatrophy illustrated here resulted from the injection of insulin. This side effect can sometimes be avoided by use of a single-peak insulin preparation. Atrophy of tissue may follow injection into it of many materials. For example, deposition of corticosteroids often causes temporary atrophy. Localized lipoatrophy may sometimes occur in patients with a number of different autoimmune diseases, and it occurs very rarely as an isolated finding in the otherwise healthy child.

Figure 616

Lipoatrophy (lipodystrophy)   Progressive lipoatrophy is characterized by the loss of all adipose tissue in the upper portion of the body. Patients characteristically have the emaciated "sunken-cheek" appearance that is seen in Fig. 616. A frequent complication of progressive lipoatrophy is membranoprolilferative glomerulonephritis, associated with decreased levels of the third component of complement. A majority of patients are female.

Figure 617

Acanthosis nigricans and lipoatrophy   Patients with either partial lipodystrophy or congenital total lipodystrophy may develop severe acanthosis nigricans. Note the severity of acanthosis nigricans in this young patient. The congenital form of lipodystrophy evolves during the first 2 years of life and is inherited in autosomal recessive fashion. Other features include insulin-resistant diabetes mellitus and accelerated growth. This combination may be referred to as the Lawrence-Seip-Berardinelli syndrome.

20

Vascular and Lymphatic Dysplasias

Figure 618

Cutis marmorata This title means ''marbled skin'' and is intended to describe the appearance of skin in which the terminal vessels are so superficial and dilated that they are constantly visible in patterns that vaguely suggest veined marble. This condition is physiologic in the newborn and represents a vasomotor response to lowering of the environmental temperature. Persistent cutis marmorata is seen in Down's syndrome and in trisomy 18.

Figure 619

Cutis marmorata telangiectatica congenita (phlebectasia congenita) This condition is present at birth and consists of accentuated vascular markings (cutis marmorata), along with areas of telangiectasia, ulceration, and atrophy. The lesions may be localized or generalized. A significant number of children with this condition have other abnormalities, among them mental retardation and hemiatrophy or hemihypertrophy. The mottling improves gradually with age in most patients.

Figure 620

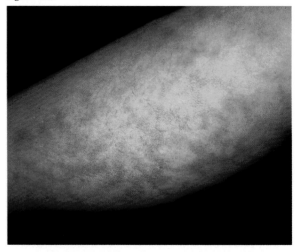

Livedo reticularis *Livedo* means a slate-gray blueness. *Reticularis* means like a net. The term describes a network of gray-blueness that is generally seen on the lower extremities. The idiopathic form of this disorder, most common in young women, carries a good prognosis. However, livedo reticularis is also seen in association with polyarteritis nodosa, systemic lupus erythematosus, and cryoglobulinemia.

Figure 621

Angioma serpiginosum This rare vascular disorder is most commonly seen in girls and tends to favor the extremities. The patient shown has numerous areas of vascular ectasia in a gyrate pattern. As one observes the condition over long periods of time, one sees resolution of old lesions and development of new ones at the periphery. While the condition tends to improve, it never quite leaves.

Figure 622

Figure 623

Salmon patch The salmon patch is by far the most common vascular lesion in the newborn. This midline or symmetrical pink macular lesion is most commonly seen on the eyelids, the nape of the neck, and the glabella. The last two are commonly described as ''stork bite'' and ''angel's kiss,'' respectively. The glabellar lesion in Fig. 622 can be expected to resolve spontaneously, as do lesions on the eyelids. Rarely, a salmon patch on the neck may persist into adult life.

Port-wine stain This unilateral vascular malformation has a markedly different histology, significance, and natural history from that of the salmon patch. The port-wine stain is made up of capillary ectasias that may be present throughout the dermis and that gradually increase with age. The color changes from pink to purple as the patient grows, and the lesions may become nodular during adult life. Because port-wine stains show no tendency to involute, they may represent a significant, lifelong cosmetic problem.

Figure 624

Figure 625

Port-wine stain In Fig. 624 we see the kind of port-wine stain that is a serious cosmetic hardship. Previous therapeutic approaches, including surgery, dermabrasion, tattooing, and use of the argon laser have met with poor-to-variable results. The tunable pulsed dye laser is a considerably more successful modality in the treatment of disfiguring port-wine stains. Success is related to the fact that hemoglobin preferentially absorbs laser energy at the 577-nm wavelength. The very

brief pulse duration prevents the heat from spreading from the blood vessels into the surrounding connective tissue. Therefore, the danger of scarring is minimized. Shown in Fig. 625 is a relatively small port-wine stain that has a small papule of angiomatosis on it. Both of these patients would be excellent candidates for treatment with the pulsed dye laser.

Figure 626

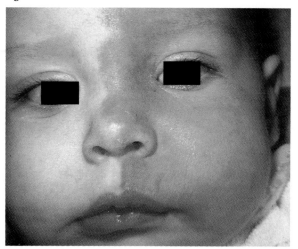

The Sturge-Weber syndrome This is one of the most serious of the angiopathies because more than merely skin is involved with the excess of blood vessels. In the case shown, deep structures (namely, the eye and meninges) have extensive vascular reduplication. The result here is glaucoma and a seizure disorder. The association between port-wine stain, seizures, and glaucoma only occurs when skin involvement includes the forehead and upper eyelid (ophthalmic or V1 trigeminal area).

Figure 627

Hemangioma Hemangiomas occur in a variety of sizes, locations, and degrees of combination of capillaries, larger vessels, and venous lakes. The one pictured here is of the simplest sort. It is limited, superficial, and largely capillary. Lesions of this sort tend to increase in size for a period of time and then to involute partially or totally. Most often, the best cosmetic result is achieved by allowing this spontaneous process to run its course.

Figure 628

Hemangioma The hemangioma illustrated is not serious in itself; it will eventually resolve spontaneously. There is, however, a danger in so young a child if the lesion should grow and mechanically close the eye. There may then be a failure of development of the cerebral area that receives visual stimuli for interpretation. This could result in ambylopia ex anopsia, a blindness from disuse. Treatment with a course of oral prednisone is indicated in such a case. The use of intralesional steroids has been advocated by some.

Figure 629

Hemangioma This picture is a good illustration of how a hemangioma resolves spontaneously. After a year or so of development, most hemangiomas begin to thrombose, and some ulcerate. Repeated events of this sort diminish the vascular bulk until nothing more than some telangiectasia, atrophy, or redundancy of overlying skin remains. Frequently no additional treatment is needed, but if necessary, minor plastic surgery is all that is required for an acceptable cosmetic result.

Figure 630

Figure 631

Hemangioma These are illustrations of a hemangioma at the height of its development on a labium majus and in almost complete spontaneous resolution. No treatment had been applied. If one could have followed the events of such a case from recognizable beginnings to end points, one would have seen originally a bit of redness, then a flowering of the lesion to the extent pictured in Fig. 630 about 1 or 1½ years later,

and finally, in the course of 2, 3, or 4 more years, the condition shown in Fig. 631. Perhaps at the very end, nothing more than some macular telangiectasia or some redundancy of skin would remain. In a site like this, whatever remains could be left alone. Serial photographs of this sort may be reassuring to the parents of a child with a hemangioma.

Figure 632

Figure 633

Disseminated hemangiomatosis Pictured here is a neonate with multiple small hemangiomas. Children with this degree of cutaneous involvement may suffer from visceral hemangiomatosis. Liver, spleen, lungs, and the gastrointestinal and central nervous systems may be involved. Risks include high-output congestive heart failure, thrombocytopenia, and neurological complications. If a complete workup establishes the presence of extensive visceral disease, early corticosteroid therapy is advisable.

Pyogenic granuloma This is a common, acquired lesion which develops at the site of an obvious or unnoticed trauma. It is the result of a local vascular proliferation. Typically, a pyogenic granuloma grows rapidly, and there is often a history of spontaneous bleeding. The lesion is usually a red papule or nodule the size of a of small nut, and it can be located anywhere on the body. Treatment consists of thorough electrodesiccation and curettage.

Figure 634

Figure 635

Glomus tumor Vascular shunts are special structures abundant in acral parts of the body that have large area and relatively small volume, like the fingertips, nose, and the pinnae of ears. They are much sparser elsewhere. Their function is to alter circulation under the stimulus of cold in such a manner as to conserve heat by turning off much of arterial circulation. Their structure is of a myoepithelium, i.e., a conglomeration of epithelial cells that have contractile ability. Such tissue sometimes becomes benignly hyperplastic

and somewhat bulky. The purplish nodule in Fig. 634 is typical of the glomus tumor. Solitary glomus tumors are often located in the nail bed, as in Fig. 635, and may give rise to severe episodes of paroxysmal pain. The subungual lesions seem to be more common in females. Excision of painful lesions is the treatment of choice. In addition, a rare syndrome of multiple glomus tumors exists. These lesions tend to be asymptomatic, and the condition is inherited in autosomal dominant fashion.

Figure 636

Figure 637

Histopathology of superficial and cavernous hemangiomas These vascular harmartomas are cellular angiomas in which one finds almost confluent sheets of proliferating endothelial cells; small, well-formed vascular channels (illustrated here); and at times somewhat larger (cavernous) vessels. Whatever the clinical and histologic pictures, they are all the same in their embryonic dysgenesis and in their strong tendency to eventual spontaneous resolution.

Histopathology of glomus tumors Glomangiomas are uncommon vascular tumors, usually acral, solitary, and tender, but at times multiple, asymptomatic, and scattered. The solitary ones tend to be highly cellular; the multiple tend to be cavernous. In addition to the endothelial-lined vessels, there is a proliferation in the form of sheets of cells that are contractile like smooth muscle cells. They have round nuclei and resemble epithelial cells. Tenderness is probably produced by contraction of these cells and stimulation of nerve fibers.

Figure 638

Figure 639

Angiokeratoma (Mibelli) There are many forms of neoangiogenesis that are benign. Pyogenic granuloma, nevus araneus, and ruby spots are examples. Angiokeratoma (Mibelli) is another type that is distinguished by the development of hyperkeratosis on small papular angiomas. The feet and lower extremities are common sites for this condition. These lesions arise during adolescence and may be associated with cold intolerance. Papular lesions of the same sort are common on the scrotum, where hyperkeratosis does not develop. These are sometimes labeled *angiokeratoma of Fordyce*. At first glance, one might think the condition as illustrated may be verruca vulgaris. Biopsy distinguishes with certainty.

Figure 640

Figure 641

Solitary angiokeratoma This lesion usually develops on the lower extremities, sometimes in response to trauma. The lesion pictured here could easily be mistaken for a melanoma or a pigmented basal cell carcinoma. Biopsy is indicated, and the combination of dilated blood vessels, hyperkeratosis, and acanthosis enables the dermatopathologist to make the correct diagnosis. When lesions of this type enlarge to the size of a plaque, the term *angiokeratoma circumscriptum* is used.

Fabry's disease (angiokeratoma corporis diffusum) This condition is serious because it is a sphingolipoidosis associated with an enzyme anomaly that leads to the deposition of a ceramide hexoside in the smooth muscle of blood vessels. The cutaneous lesions are tiny papules that are angiomatous. When this happens in the blood vessels of the heart, kidneys, eyes, and nervous system, symptoms of functional disturbance and failure appear. Fucosidosis and sialidosis may cause a similar clinical appearance.

Figure 642

Figure 643

Hereditary hemorrhagic telangiectasia (Osler-Rendu-Weber syndrome) This is an autosomal dominant syndrome with both cutaneous and visceral involvement. In most children with the disease, the presenting symptom is recurrent epistaxis. Patients go on to develop vascular papules that stud the lips, tongue, palate, and nasal mucosa. The ears, palms, soles, digital tips, and nail beds are other common sites for lesions. As the disease progresses, melena and hematemesis may develop as a result of gastrointestinal involvement. A significant number of patients with this syndrome have hepatic and pulmonary arteriovenous fistulas. The latter may lead to cyanosis, shortness of breath, polycythemia and digital clubbing. Patients must be monitored carefully for hemorrhage in the liver, brain, urinary bladder, and retina and for the development of a secondary anemia.

Figure 644

Figure 645

Histopathology of Fabry's disease Fabry's disease (angiokeratoma corporis diffusum) is histologically classed among the angiokeratomas, i.e., hemangiomas that show a variable degree of surface hyperkeratosis. It is known to be caused by an inborn error of metabolism (a specific, heritable enzyme defect). Microscopically, one sees cavernous, endothelium-lined blood vessels directly beneath a thinned epidermis. There is no hyperkeratosis visible in this figure. The microscopic picture is typical, but not unique.

Spider angioma (nevus araneus) This is a trivial and common childhood angioma, highly characteristic in its central vascular punctum from which radiate fine vessels that give the entire lesion the fanciful appearance of a spider in its web. Such lesions are usually solitary, and the face is a common site for them. The dorsa of the hands are another common site. Persistent lesions are easily extirpated by skillful electrodesiccation or by the use of the tunable pulsed dye laser.

Figure 646

Figure 647

Klippel-Trenaunay-Weber syndrome This is a condition in which hemangiomas, varicosities, and phlebectasia cover an entire limb or other body area. There may be associated skeletal abnormalities, including macrodactyly and syndactyly. A combination of port-wine stain and hemangiomas may be present from birth. The osteohypertrophy develops during the first several years of life. The photographs are front and back views of an infant who has the beginning of the angiomatous process. At this stage, the condition appears almost like a nevus flammeus. Over time, more massive vascularization and enlargement of the limb will develop.

Figure 648

Figure 649

Milroy's disease This term refers to a form of primary lymphedema that is inherited in autosomal dominant fashion. The swelling of the feet and legs is either unilateral or bilateral. The edema is pitting at first, but fibrosis of the lower extremities gradually leads to a firmer and more persistent enlargement. Over time, the overlying epidermis may become verrucous and hyperkeratotic.

Lymphangioma The proliferation of lymphatic channels in the skin or subcutaneous tissue may give rise to lesions with a variety of clinical appearance. Most lymphangiomas develop during the first 2 years of life, and some are present at birth. The cluster of clear vesicles pictured here is termed *lymphangioma circumscriptum*. The lesions are benign but may be distressing because of their tendency to increase in size and number over time and to occasionally become irritated or superinfected.

Figure 650

Figure 651

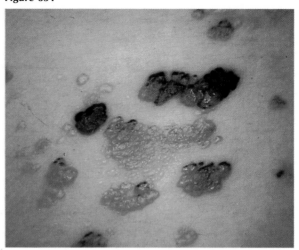

Lymphangioma (cont.)   Illustrated in these two photographs are additional examples of lymphangioma circumscriptum. Figure 650 shows why the appearance of these glistening papules is sometimes compared to frog spawn. Figure 651 is a mixed hamartoma composed of both lymphatic channels and blood vessels. The surgical treatment of lymphangioma

circumscriptum is complicated by the fact that the associated lymphatic channels may be deeper than can be clinically appreciated. The result is a high rate of recurrence. Laser surgery may be a reasonable approach for some of these lesions.

Figure 652

Figure 653

Lymphangioma   Lymphangioma circumscriptum is usually localized to the neck, proximal extremities, abdomen, tongue, and mucous membranes. The lesion pictured here is in an unusual location. The surface is hyperkeratotic, and one can imagine confusing this lymphangioma with a large verruca. Plastic surgery would possibly yield a good result in a localized, easily accessible lesion like this one.

Histopathology of lymphangioma   Lymphangiomas consist of proliferating, thin-walled lymphatic channels. They are commonly superficial, though frequently a deep component is also present, which accounts for recurrence when destruction of what is merely visible is practiced. In the photomicrograph, one sees, just beneath the epidermis, vessels that contain pink proteinaceous material. The contents of vessels in histologic sections cannot always be relied on to distinguish lymphatics from blood vessels.

21

Neoplastic Diseases

Figure 654

Leukemia cutis A dermal infiltrate of leukemic cells results in the papulonodular lesions, or plaques, which are illustrated here. Such primary involvement of the skin is relatively rare in childhood leukemia. The wide variety of secondary manifestations of leukemia includes petechiae and ecchymoses and pyoderma gangrenosum. A polymorphonuclear dermal infiltrate termed *Sweet's syndrome* may be associated with leukemia. In addition, children receiving chemotherapy are prone to bacterial and fungal infections of the skin, severe varicella, and ulcerative or chronic herpes simplex.

Figure 655

Hodgkin's disease Like other lymphoproliferative disorders, Hodgkin's disease may have both specific and nonspecific cutaneous manifestations. Figure 655 illustrates a relatively rare event in children with Hodgkin's disease: the direct infiltration of malignant cells into the skin. A biopsy of these brownish papules, nodules, and plaques reveals a histology similar to that of affected lymph nodes. These lesions may occasionally ulcerate, and pruritus is a distressing symptom.

Figure 656

Neuroblastoma, metastatic This malignant tumor of the autonomic nervous system occurs most frequently in young children. Metastatic disease is very often present at the time of diagnosis. Cutaneous metastases appear as bluish papules or nodules involving the trunk or extremities. They are sometimes noted to blanch upon stroking and may sometimes exhibit increased sweating. Children who are under the age of 1 year at the time of diagnosis often experience spontaneous regression of their illness. The prognosis in older children and in those with very widespread disease tends to be poor.

Figure 657

Histopathology of metastatic neuroblastoma In the neonatal period, neuroblastoma is the most common condition that metastasizes to the skin. This does not in itself portend a grave prognosis. The cells spread to the skin hematogenously from the primary neoplasm. Microscopically the diagnosis is easily established if one finds the typical rosettes so well illustrated in the figure. Nuclei are arranged in a peripheral palisade about a central area of cellular material that, but for the rosettes, could be misinterpreted as fibrin.

Figure 658

Figure 659

Histiocytosis X This is a spectrum of disease which encompasses Letterer-Siwe disease, Hand-Schüller-Christian disease, and eosinophilic granuloma. The disorder is characterized by the proliferation of Langerhans histioctyes in the skin and other organ systems. Figure 658 shows the characteristic seborrheic-like scaly, erythematous eruption on the scalp, face, and ears. A similar eruption, accompanied by erosive and granulomatous changes, may be seen in the neck folds, as in Fig. 659, or in the axillae and diaper area. In general,

an unusual or recalcitrant diaper rash of this general appearance should alert the physician to consider the diagnosis. The presence of petechiae is a particularly helpful sign. Diagnosis is confirmed by skin biopsy (Fig. 661). More rapid confirmation is sometimes possible by observing the presence of histiocytes in a lesion that has been scraped onto a microscopic slide and stained. Histiocytosis X may be accompanied by hepatosplenomegaly, lymphadenopathy, anemia, and thrombocytopenia.

Figure 660

Figure 661

Histiocytosis X The child shown here is covered with numerous red-brown, crusted papules, which may become hemorrhagic. Rarely, this clinical picture is present at birth. The prognosis of children with histiocytosis X is extremely variable but is certainly worse in patients who develop organ dysfunction from their disease. The decision to initiate chemotherapy should be based on the clinical course of the individual patient.

Histopathology of histiocytosis X The diagnosis of histiocytosis X is established by biopsy of a skin lesion. Microscopically one finds a dermal infiltrate of large, rounded histiocytes with abundant eosinophilic cytoplasm. The abnormal cells may invade the epidermis. The eccentrically located nuclei are typically kidney-shaped and may be large and hyperchromatic. Electron microscopic examination is sometimes used to confirm the diagnosis. The abnormal histiocytes in areas of involvement are noted to contain so-called Langerhans granules in their cytoplasm.

22

Adnexal Dysplasias

Figure 662

Figure 663

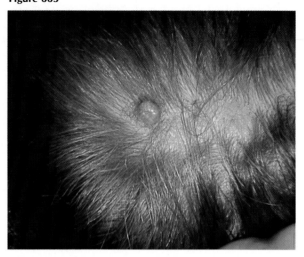

Nevus sebaceus This is a hamartoma composed of sebaceous glands. It usually presents at birth as a yellow nodule or pebbled, hairless plaque on the scalp, forehead, or neck. The photograph in Fig. 662 shows the color and shape of the congenital lesion. With the loss of the effect of maternal hormones during the first few months of life, the lesion may quickly flatten and lose its distinctive color. During puberty, the nevus sebaceus again becomes raised, yellow, and ver-

rucous. After this change, and usually during adulthood, nevus sebaceus may give rise to a wide variety of benign and malignant neoplasms. These include basal cell hamartomas, keratoacanthomas, syringocystadenoma papilliferum, basal cell epitheliomas, and, rarely, squamous cell carcinomas. Figure 663 shows a basal cell carcinoma that has developed on a plaque of nevus sebaceus.

Figure 664

Figure 665

Nevus sebaceus Here pictured is another nevus sebaceus on which basal cell carcinoma has developed. In this case the color appears more brown and blackish in the main lesion, but the yellow color can still be appreciated in the small outlying papules. The nodule near the center represents the malignant change. Because neoplasms eventually occur in about one-third of patients with nevus sebaceus, it is considered advisable to arrange for the excision of all such lesions before puberty.

Histopathology of nevus sebaceus This is a localized cutaneous dysplasia in which disordered structure involves the epidermis, cutaneous appendages, and dermis. In the illustration one sees a rugose, hyperplastic epidermis; sebaceous glands without hair follicles; and cystic sweat gland elements (presumably apocrine) on the left. The impression gained is of a flawed attempt to form normal structures. Basal-cell epithelioma and a variety of adnexal neoplasms develop in a nevus sebaceus.

Figure 666

Figure 667

Syringoma These very small papules are adenomas of intraepidermal eccrine ducts. Most commonly, syringomas develop on the eyelids of women during adolescence or early adult life. Figure 666 is a good example of the fine papules that occur on the lower eyelids. They have no malignant potential, but the lesions are usually multiple, and therefore the cause of cosmetic concern. Syringomas of this type may

be delicately removed by electrodesiccation and curettage. Figure 667 is a representation of even smaller lesions, this time on the upper part of the chest. Rarely, a child or adolescent will develop successive crops of syringomas on the skin of the anterior neck, antecubital fossa, axilla, and groin. This condition, termed *eruptive syringoma,* is sometimes inherited in autosomal dominant fashion.

Figure 668

Figure 669

Histopathology of syringomas Syringomas are the most common malformations of cutaneous appendanges. The microscopic picture is essentially the same in the common periorbital and the rare disseminated variety. One sees numerous epithelial elements in the form of solid cords and tubules containing pink secretory material situated in dense, relatively acellular stroma.

Clear cell hidradenoma This benign eccrine sweat gland tumor occurs as a solitary lesion in most cases. Most commonly, the growth appears as a small intraepidermal nodule. Ulceration or discharge of serous material rarely occurs. The lesion is harmless and may be extirpated by shaving it off level with the surrounding skin and electrodesiccating the base.

Figure 670

Figure 671

Dermoid cyst   These lesions present in the newborn as soft, round, subcutaneous tumors that are freely movable beneath the overlying epidermis. They represent ectodermal hamartomas and occur at the site of closure of embryonic clefts. The vast majority of dermoid cysts are found near the lateral eyebrow or on the forehead. The neck is the second most common location. The lesion pictured in Fig. 670 has pro-

truding hairs and was present at birth. In Fig. 671 there is a typical mass just lateral to the eyebrow. Histologic examination of these lesions reveals combinations of epidermis, dermis, sweat glands, sebaceous glands, and hair. Surgical excision is required when the dermoid cyst interferes with closure of the eyelid and is sometimes desirable for cosmetic reasons.

Figure 672

Figure 673

Histopathology of dermoid cysts   Dermoid cysts probably result from defective fusion of embryonic structures, most commonly on the face. When in the midline of the nose, a tuft of hairs commonly emerges from a sinus. The cyst itself is lined with stratified squamous epithelium, usually with sebaceous glands and hair follicles in continuity, opening into a cyst lumen, as seen here. Sweat ducts are present less commonly; abundant smooth muscle is sometimes found.

Eccrine poroma   This is a solitary benign tumor which is most common in adults but is occasionally seen in adolescents. Eccrine poromas are usually located on the sole of the foot, although they may rarely occur in a variety of other areas. The vascular appearance of the lesion, as shown in the illustration, could lead to confusion with pyogenic granuloma. Treatment consists of complete surgical excision.

Figure 674

Figure 675

Pilomatricoma (benign calcifying epithelioma of Malherbe)
This solitary benign tumor arises most commonly during childhood, usually on the face or upper extremities. Pilomatricomas range in size from 0.5 to 3.0 cm, although they are occasionally even larger. They appear as hard, freely movable dermal nodules. The skin overlying the lesion is usually normal but is sometimes erythematous or bluish. The overlying surface may feel irregular and exhibit a "tent sign." Pilomatricoma is very rarely associated with myotonic muscular dystrophy.

Histopathology of pilomatricoma This lesion is a solid tumor that clinically simulates an epidermoid cyst. Histologically it shows differentiation like that of the matrix of a hair bulb and hence is also called *pilomatricoma*. At the lower left of the photomicrograph one sees some undifferentiated basaloid cells, but most of the tumor is composed of sheets of so-called ghost or shadow cells. Calcification, usually present, is not seen here; even ossification occasionally occurs.

Figure 676

Figure 677

Epidermal cyst The lesions that were long termed *sebaceous cysts* are now renamed *epidermal cysts* because their points of origin are not the sebaceous glands and their content is not purely sebum. Epidermal cysts are exceedingly common lesions on the face and trunk. They consist of an epithelium-lined cavity that is filled with a caseous mixture of lipid and proteinaceous matter. They may have no apparent opening onto the surface of the skin, as in Fig. 676, or they may have

a small aperture, as in Fig. 677. They may be as small as large seeds or as large as good-sized nuts. Uncomplicated epidermal cysts may be surgically removed in toto by clean dissection. They frequently become secondarily infected, and then incision and repeated drainage are required for their cure. They have no malignant potential, but sooner or later require attention because of size, location, or secondary infection.

Figure 678

Figure 679

Trichoepithelioma Trichoepithelioma is a benign neoplasm which differentiates toward hair structures. Lesions of this type may be multiple or solitary. Figure 678 illustrates a patient with multiple trichoepitheliomas. Individuals with this condition have numerous firm, rounded, skin-colored papules which are located mainly near the nasolabial folds. In more extensive cases, the rest of the face may become involved.

The lesions usually begin to emerge during puberty, and the tendency for them to develop is inherited in autosomal dominant fashion. Figure 679 shows a solitary trichoepithelioma. These single flesh-colored papules develop on the face during childhood or adolescence. Solitary trichoepitheliomas are usually not hereditary.

Figure 680

Eruptive vellus hair cysts This condition is characterized by the rapid appearance of numerous small pigmented and flesh-colored papules. The tiny dome-shaped lesions are usually clustered on the chest but may also involve the proximal extremities, buttocks, and back. The onset of this asympto-matic condition usually occurs during mid-childhood. Biopsy of a lesion reveals a mid-dermal cyst containing laminated keratinous material. Autosomal dominant inheritance of this condition is sometimes observed. Spontaneous resolution frequently occurs.

23

Benign and Malignant Pigmented Lesions

Figure 681

Figure 682

Ephelis This is the learned word for a freckle. The plural is *ephelides* (pronounced ĕf-ĕl'ĭ-dēz). These are small, brown macules that are exceedingly common on the face in some children. They appear after exposure to sunlight and are more common in children with very fair skin or red hair. They tend to disappear in adult life. Histologically, these lesions show increased amounts of epidermal melanin but no abundance of melanocytes.

Lentigo This tan-to-brown to almost brown-black macular lesion may be found on any area of the body surface, which includes mucous membranes. There is no relation to ultraviolet light exposure. The illustration is of lentigines on the lip. Lentigines may be present at birth and tend to increase in number during childhood and adult life. Histologically, there is a proliferation of melanocytes and elongation of the rete ridges. Lesions of this sort show no tendency to resolve spontaneously.

Figure 683

Figure 684

Peutz-Jeghers syndrome This autosomal dominant syndrome is notable for highly characteristic lentigines seen on the vermilion of the lips and adjacent skin, on the buccal mucosa, and on the palmar aspect of the fingertips. The pictures here are good representations of the lentigines in a typical case. Patients with this syndrome may also have gastrointestinal

polyps throughout the GI tract but most frequently in the jejunum. These benign hamartomas have very little malignant potential but may be the cause of obstruction, diarrhea, bleeding, or intussusception. Unlike common lentigines, the cutaneous lesions in these patients tend to fade during adult life. Mucous membrane lesions persist.

Figure 685

Multiple lentigines syndrome   This autosomal dominant syndrome features numerous small lentigines, which are present at or soon after birth and cover the entire cutaneous surface. The possibilities of organ involvement are summed up in the mnemonic word *leopard*, in which *l* stands for lentigines, *e* for electrocardiographic conduction defects, *o* for ocular hypertelorism, *p* for pulmonary stenosis, *a* for abnormalities of genitalia, *r* for retardation of growth, and *d* for deafness.

Figure 686

Nevocellular nevus (junction type)   The macule of hyperpigmentation here pictured is the most common form of nevocellular nevus in childhood. The so-called junction nevus is a benign lesion that is composed of melanocytic nevus cells along the dermoepidermal junction. Lesions of this sort may arise in crops after the first year of life. As nevus cells migrate into the dermis, the typical junction nevus becomes a compound nevus. This process usually occurs during adolescence and early adulthood.

Figure 687

Nevus spilus   This is a solitary flat area of light-brown pigmentation which may vary in size from 2 to 25 cm. Illustrated here is the tendency for numerous brown or black freckles of pigmentation to develop on top of the larger and lighter-colored macule. Nevus spilus should not be confused with either a congenital melanocytic nevus or a café-au-lait spot. It carries no particular malignant potential, and no treatment is required.

Figure 688

Dysplastic nevus   Nevi that show an irregular mixture of tan, black, brown, and pink and feature an uneven border are termed *dysplastic nevi*. The central portion may be darker and slightly elevated. The premalignant potential of a solitary dysplastic-appearing nevus is controversial. However, it is widely recognized that patients with a family history of melanoma and those who have numerous dysplastic nevi should be observed carefully. Individuals with the so-called dysplastic nevus syndrome are at higher risk for developing melanoma.

Figure 689

Figure 690

Compound nevus The ordinary mole has great variety in intensity of brown color, size, shape, and location. The ones termed *compound* are composed of melanocytes that are gathered into thèques or nests at the dermoepidermal junction and in larger, less compact collections deeper in the dermis. Shown in Fig. 689 is a plaque that is light brown and of fairly large size as compound nevi go; Figure 690 shows a papule that is reddish-brown and of a more usual size. Such lesions are thought to start out as junction nevi, which then go on

to more melanocytic proliferation; melanocytes continue to drop off and down, becoming collections in the dermis. At any time in the development of compound nevi, melanocytes are found both at the dermoepidermal junction and in the dermis. Generally speaking, these lesions are benign and remain so. If cosmetically objectionable, they may be excised in toto or shaved off. Histologic examination of all surgically removed pigmented lesions is advisable.

Figure 691

Figure 692

Intradermal nevus The illustrations here are of common moles in which the collections of melanocytes are entirely intradermal. Such lesions do not show any thèques or nests of melanocytes at the dermoepidermal junction. They too come in a great variety of colors, shapes, sizes, and sites. Intradermal nevi are the end stage of development of junction

and compound nevi. As with junction and compound nevi, they are extremely common and benign. Like compound nevi, they may be ablated by shaving or elliptical excision. Treatment by these methods does not increase the possibility of malignant transformation.

Figure 693

Figure 694

Histopathology of compound and intradermal nevi The precursors of the pigment-producing cells (melanocytes) migrate early in fetal development from the neural crest through the mesenchyme to the epidermis, where they normally remain in the basal (germinative) layer in functional harmony with the more numerous keratinocytes. About every sixth cell in the basal layer is a melanocyte. The melanin that melanocytes produce is transferred by dendrites to neaby keratinocytes. Should melanocytes proliferate but remain with the epidermis, a so-called junction (intraepidermal) nevus forms. The proliferating cells generally gather into nests (thèques) at the tips of rete ridges. If some of these cells "drop" into the dermis, a compound nevus (illustrated on the left) develops. When intraepidermal proliferation of melanocytes ceases and all of them come to be in the corium (illustrated on the right), the nevus is designated *intradermal*.

Figure 695

Figure 696

Halo nevus This is a relatively common condition in which an area of depigmentation develops around an existing melanocytic nevus. Lesions of this type, also termed *leukoderma acquisitum centrifugum*, are not unusual during childhood. They may be single or multiple. Figure 695 shows a small halo around a typical compound nevus. Over time, the nevus itself may depigment (Fig. 696) and disappear, and the skin color of the entire area may return to normal. The development of a halo around a nevus is probably due to an immune response to the melanocytes of the original lesion. Halo nevi are more common in children with vitiligo and have been very rarely seen in association with malignant melanoma at another site. For most halo nevi, no treatment is required. When biopsy is performed, there is a dense lymphohistiocytic infiltrate around the central pigmented lesion.

Figure 697

Figure 698

Spitz nevus This completely benign melanocytic lesion most often occurs during childhood. Spitz nevi are usually solitary, dome-shaped papules or nodules. They frequently arise on the face and extremities. The red-to-red-brown color of the papular lesions in Fig. 697 and Fig. 698 is fairly typical. Occasionally, they may be flesh-colored or brown-black.

There is often a history of rapid growth. There is little data on the natural history of these lesions, but the customary treatment consists of a conservative complete excision. Rarely, patients may develop multiple Spitz nevi. These multiple and agminated Spitz nevi may occur over a large café-au-lait spot.

Figure 699

Figure 700

Histopathology of Spitz nevus Spitz nevus, formerly termed *benign juvenile melanoma,* is felt by most dermatopathologists to be a form of compound nevus. The presence of pleomorphism, numerous mitotic figures, and a dense inflammatory cell infiltrate may at times suggest the diagnosis of nodular malignant melanoma. Before the historic work of the late Dr. Sophie Spitz, many such lesions were, in fact,

misdiagnosed as melanoma. Dr. Spitz defined a typical architecture and cell morphology that are associated with a good prognosis. Pictured in Fig. 699 is the nest of large, epithelioid cells, which are typical of this lesion. Spindle cells, the other cell population in Spitz nevus, are shown in Fig. 700. Such lesions have also been termed *spindle-* and *epithelioid-cell nevi.*

Figure 701

Congenital melanocytic nevus   This pigmented lesion is present at birth in about 1 percent of all infants. The typical appearance is a flat tan or brown macule of irregular shape. The lesion may be studded with fine papules or may even be nodular. As illustrated here, a congenital melanocytic nevus may develop numerous coarse hairs. Biopsy of a lesion reveals nevus cells in the deep dermis between collagen bundles and adjacent to adnexae. Because the true incidence of malignant melanoma arising in small congenital melanocytic nevi is uncertain, management remains controversial.

Figure 702

Congenital melanocytic nevus   The lesion shown here is surrounded by a border of depigmentation. The occurrence of a halo congenital melanocytic nevus is fairly unusual. The spontaneous regression of a portion of a pigmented lesion is probably due to a host antibody response to a subset of melanocytes. This phenomenon is sometimes associated with the development of melanoma. However, in most cases, the formation of such a halo is a benign event. Complete and spontaneous resolution of even very large congenital melanocytic nevi may occur.

Figure 703

Congenital melanocytic nevus   A congenital melanocytic nevus may cover large parts of the cutaneous surface. A lesion in the distribution illustrated here is sometimes referred to as a bathing trunk nevus. The possibility of malignant melanoma developing within such a large congenital melanocytic nevus represents a significant problem. Varying studies estimate the incidence of this occurrence somewhere between

Figure 704

6 and 36 percent. Therefore, the excision of giant congenital melanocytic nevi is recommended whenever feasible. The use of inflatable tissue expanders enables the surgeon to remove large portions of lesions like this one without skin grafting. Patients with congenital melanocytic nevi on the scalp or mid-back must also be investigated for the possibility of leptomeningeal melanocytosis or other neurologic defects.

Figure 705

Figure 706

Malignant melanoma Less than 2 percent of all melanomas occur during childhood. Nonetheless, attention must be paid to signs and symptoms suggestive of this potentially fatal disease. Variegations of color are of particular concern. Irregular or notched borders, bleeding and ulceration are other signs of malignant change. The patient may give a history of itching, and the parents may have noted rapid growth of the lesion. Because the prognosis of a melanoma is most closely related to the thickness of the lesion at the time of treatment, emphasis should be on early diagnosis.

Histopathology of malignant melanoma Three types of melanoma may occur in children: superficial spreading, nodular, and acral lentiginous. The commonest is the superficial spreading variety, pictured in Fig. 706. The photomicrograph shows nests of atypical melanocytes lying at all levels of the epidermis. These tumors may have a long phase of radial growth in the epidermis and at the dermoepidermal junction. Eventually, penetration into the dermis occurs, with a rapid worsening of prognosis. Measurements of tumor depth are used to establish prognosis and appropriate therapy.

Figure 707

Figure 708

Mongolian spot This very common cutaneous lesion is caused by a collection of melanocytes scattered through the deep dermis. The sacral location in Fig. 707 is by far the most frequent, but dermal melanosis may be present in other areas as well. Mongolian spots are found in many black newborns but are significantly less common among white infants. The areas of blue-gray pigmentation are usually present at birth and almost always fade during the first years of life.

Blue nevus Collections of melanocytes deep in the dermis produce a blue macule or papule such as that illustrated. The physics of color in the skin is such that melanin high in the dermis makes for black coloration, lower in the dermis, blue. Blue nevi are small dome-shaped nodules that are often located on the dorsa of the hands or feet. They frequently arise during childhood. The common blue nevus has no potential for malignancy. Malignant degeneration of a cellular blue nevus occurs rarely.

Figure 709

Figure 710

Nevus of Ota This rare dyschromia is characterized by a persistent bluish-gray discoloration of the skin around the eye. The proliferation of melanocytes in the upper dermis may extend to the forehead, malar area, and nose. Ocular involvement always includes the sclera, as in this patient, and sometimes the iris, conjunctiva, and optic nerve. Nevus of Ota is considered a benign dermatosis, but melanoma on the ipsilateral side has been known to occur.

Nevus of Ito The occurrence of a pathological process identical to nevus of Ota, on the skin of the deltoid, scapular, and clavicular regions, is termed *nevus of Ito*. The color tends to be somewhat browner than the mongolian spot, because of the distribution of melanocytes higher in the dermis. In contrast to the mongolian spot, these lesions tend to persist through adult life.

Figure 711

Becker's nevus This lesion is an irregular, pigmented macule which most commonly arises in boys at puberty. The light-brown area of pigmentation, which may be quite large, eventually develops thick hairs. The most typical location for Becker's nevus is on the shoulder or upper back. Less commonly, lesions arise on the forearm, upper chest, and abdomen. Becker's nevus has no malignant potential, and, therefore, surgical removal is not necessary. The pigmentation and hypertrichosis both tend to persist into adult life.

24

Miscellaneous Pigmentary Disorders

Figure 712

Incontinentia pigmenti This rare condition is characterized by linear and whorled lesions and a wide variety of systemic manifestations. Incontinentia pigmenti is inherited as an X-linked dominant trait and is seen almost exclusively in girls. The cutaneous eruption is usually present at birth and evolves through three stages. Lesions typical of the first two stages, vesicular and verrucous, are seen in Fig. 712. Over several

Figure 713

months the raised areas flatten, and the patient is left with widespread whorled, or ''marble-cake,'' hyperpigmentation, as pictured in Fig. 713. In turn, the lesions of this third, hyperpigmented stage fade over a period of several years. The disorder may also result in scarring alopecia of the scalp, dystrophic nails, and abnormalities of the teeth.

Figure 714

Incontinentia pigmenti This illustration is a good representation of how extensive and bizarre the dyschromia of incontinentia pigmenti can be. Central nervous system and ocular abnormalities are the most serious aspects of this disease. One third of patients will develop seizures, mental retardation, or spastic paralysis. Eye involvement may include the presence of a retrolental mass, retinal detachment, cataracts, and optic atrophy. Skeletal anomalies are sometimes seen.

Figure 715

Histopathology of incontinentia pigmenti The three classic stages of incontinentia pigmenti differ histologically and clinically. The third stage, from which the condition derives its name, is microscopically the least specific. In the early vesicular stage, illustrated here, one sees intraepidermal, spongiotic blisters containing mainly eosinophils. Both this stage and the second, verrucous, stage display keratinized, eosinophilic malpighian cells, one of which is seen on the left.

Figure 716

Figure 717

Incontinentia pigmenti achromians (hypomelanosis of Ito) This condition is characterized by whorled areas of hypopigmentation which are present from birth or evolve during early childhood. The lesions may be generalized, but individual areas of hypopigmentation tend to respect the midline. A significant number of patients with this pigmentary disorder have central nervous system disease, usually manifest as seizures or mental retardation. Hypertelorism is the most common of the musculoskeletal abnormalities seen in this disorder.

Nevus depigmentosus (achromicus) These are localized areas of hypopigmentation which are usually present at birth. The lesions may be irregular in size and shape and occasionally follow a linear or segmental pattern. Electron microscopic study of these areas suggests that melanosomes are not being transferred from melanocytes into surrounding keratinocytes. There are no associated abnormalities.

Figure 718

Figure 719

Nevus anemicus This circumscribed area of macular hypopigmentation is due to a localized vascular abnormality. Chest and back are the most common locations. In contrast to nevus depigmentosus, erythema does not develop in response to stroking or the application of ice or warm water. Hypersensitivity of the involved vessels to catecholamines has been postulated as a cause.

Carotenemia The vegetable pigment carotene is widely distributed in carrots, lettuce, squash, and many other vegetables and fruits. A diet which is very rich in these foods results in a yellowish-orange discoloration of the skin. This appearance is usually localized to the palms and soles (note the hand on the left) but may also involve the skin of the face. The presence of normal sclerae distinguishes the clinical appearance of this condition from that of jaundice. Return to normal skin color follows a reduction in dietary intake of carotene.

Figure 720

Figure 721

Waardenburg's syndrome This genetic disorder is transmitted as an autosomal dominant, with variable penetrance. It is characterized grossly by partial albinism in the form of a white forelock (Fig. 720), broad nasal root (Figs. 720 and 721), hypertrichosis of the inner portions of the eyebrows, lateral displacement of the medial canthi (Figs. 720 and 721), partial or complete heterochromia of the irides (Fig. 721), and complete or unilateral deafness. In blacks, blue irides, vitiligo, and pigmentary changes in the fundi may be seen. There are no other constitutional symptoms, but the hearing loss and unusual appearance may pose handicaps.

Figure 722

Figure 723

Partial albinism (piebaldism) Patients with this autosomal dominant condition have congenital patches of depigmentation. Most have a white forelock, with involvement of adjoining scalp and forehead in a triangular pattern. There may be other areas of involvement on the trunk and extremities. Electron microscopic examination of affected areas reveals a complete absence of melanocytes. Management must include the appropriate use of sunscreen lotions on depigmented skin.

Albinism This condition is characterized by congenital hypopigmentation of the skin, hair, and eyes. Almost all of the many varieties are inherited in autosomal recessive fashion. Photophobia is a significant problem for most patients. The lack of protective melanin leads to extreme sun sensitivity and results in a high incidence of actinic keratoses, basal cell carcinomas, and squamous cell carcinomas. The avoidance of sun exposure through the use of protective clothing and sunscreen preparations is critical.

Figure 724

Figure 725

Vitiligo About half of the patients with vitiligo have onset of their disease during childhood or adolescence. Patients may present with hypopigmented and depigmented macules of various sizes and shapes. The area of involvement surrounding the eye in Fig. 724 represents one fairly typical distribution. Note the associated depigmentation of eyebrows and eyelashes. Periorificial vitiligo may also involve the skin around the mouth, rectum, and genitalia. Vitiligo may occur

only on the distal extremities or may be unilateral and segmental, as in Fig. 725. Vitiligo may be associated with uveitis and peripheral retinal scarring, but these changes rarely affect vision. The frequent presence of antibodies to melanocytes in individuals with vitiligo suggests an autoimmune etiology. A number of other autoimmune disorders, including Addison's disease and Hashimoto's thyroiditis, are more common among patients with vitiligo and their relatives.

Figure 726

Figure 727

Vitiligo These are more illustrations of fairly extensive cases of vitiligo. The condition tends to progress and may even become universal. A variety of treatment modalities are commonly employed, with varying degrees of success. The patient and family should be made aware of the sophisticated cover-up cosmetics which are now available. The use of broad-spectrum sunscreen lotions during the summer months

minimizes the contrast between normal and involved skin. For some patients, the application of topical corticosteroids early in the course of the disease may induce repigmentation. Finally, varying combinations of topical or oral psoralens and ultraviolet A light (PUVA) are used in the treatment of vitiligo.

Figure 728

Figure 729

The Chédiak-Higashi syndrome This genetic disorder, recessive in mechanism of transmission, is extremely rare. It is characterized by albinism, photophobia, lymphadenopathy, hepatosplenomegaly, and susceptibility to pyogenic infection. The peripheral blood smear reveals giant granules within lymphocytes. The high incidences of serious infection and lymphoreticular malignancy contribute to a poor prognosis.

Linea alba This linear stripe of hypopigmentation in the mid-chest and abdomen is termed *linea alba. Linea nigra* is its hyperpigmented counterpart. This is one of several locations for the extremely common and completely benign pigmentary demarcation lines. Other sites include the upper, lateral arms, the mid-posterior legs, and the central back. There may also be two symmetrical lines crossing from the mid-clavicle to the areolae.

Figure 730

Figure 731

Postinflammatory hypopigmentation A wide variety of dermatologic diseases may leave either temporary or permanent hypopigmentation. Figure 730 shows loss of pigment in the popliteal fossa of a child who has atopic dermatitis. This process results from the inflammatory disease itself and from chronic scratching. The same phenomenon is shown on the face in Fig. 731. This is probably also the result of atopic dermatitis. Postinflammatory hypopigmentation can usually be easily differentiated from vitiligo. The lesions that follow inflammatory skin disease are less well defined and are more off-white than stark white. The symmetry that may occur in vitiligo is not seen here. For most children, postinflammatory hypopigmentation is temporary. Parents should be reassured that even the most disfiguring patterns of pigmentary alteration will resolve with proper therapy and time.

25

Artifacts and Anomalies of Hair and Nails

Figure 732

Figure 733

Child abuse The physical abuse of children accounts for approximately 2000 deaths per year in the United States. Physicians who care for children must acquaint themselves with the signs of battering, sexual abuse, and nutritional deprivation. For the protection of children, the laws in all states require the reporting of all cases of suspected child abuse. Illustrated here are typical loop marks in a child who

was struck with a doubled-over rope or electrical cord. The presence of ecchymoses or scars on the lower back or buttocks is almost always the result of physical abuse. Slap marks, human bites, and lash marks each leave bruises of a distinctive shape and distribution. The presence of bruises of this sort is evidence of force without restraint and is a definite sign of child abuse.

Figure 734

Figure 735

Child abuse Ten percent of the cases of physical abuse in children involve the deliberate infliction of burns as a form of punishment. Cigarette burns, which appear as uniform round erosions, are often located on the palms and soles. Second degree burns may also occur when a child is held against a radiator or hot plate. Illustrated here are two burns which resulted from forcible immersion in hot water. Sym-

metrical blistering of the perineum (Fig. 734) is evidence of a child being lowered into a hot bath. Figure 735 is illustrative of forcible immersion of a hand. In general, the presence of an injury for which the history seems implausible should alert the physician to the possibility of child abuse. A delay in seeking medical assistance for the care of an injury should also cause concern.

Figure 736

Factitial dermatitis   Injuries to the skin that are induced by the patient or another individual are termed *factitial derma-titis*. This entity, when it occurs in childhood, may be related to a variety of emotional disturbances in either parent or child. The lesions in Fig. 736 are self-inflicted wounds caused by bites. Some are scars and others are inflammatory lesions. The distribution and morphology of lesions of this type are

Figure 737

not consistent with any known cutaneous disease, and there is usually no credible history for their development. Other methods of inducing self-injury include scratching, picking, and gouging. The hypertrichosis in Fig. 737 resulted from repeated biting on the skin in a child with severe mental retardation. Self-mutilation of this type is also seen in the Lesch-Nyhan syndrome.

Figure 738

Factitial dermatitis   Figure 738 shows ecthymatous lesions that might have been produced by fingernails. Figure 739 shows the sort of lesions caused by caustic chemicals. Self-induced injury of this sort is associated with a wide range of emotional disturbances or psychiatric disease. Healing of lesions can sometimes be facilitated by occlusion of the area of skin that is being repeatedly injured. Psychiatric referral

Figure 739

is often of value. A particular cause of factitial dermatitis in children is termed *Munchausen's-by-proxy syndrome*. In this condition, a disturbed parent attempts to create the appearance of illness in a child. The presence of this syndrome signals a high level of physical danger for the child, and cases of this sort must be promptly reported to social service agencies as a form of child abuse.

Figure 740

Figure 741

Pseudoainhum The word *ainhum* means "to saw." True ainhum is limited geographically to Africa and usually presents as a groove encircling the small toe. Pseudoainhum refers to a condition which is clinically similar but caused by a wide variety of disease processes. In children, congenital constricting bands may be a cause. More commonly, pseudoainhum occurs as an artifact from the wind of a cord or a long hair buried around a digit. In Fig. 740, the third toe is affected by a groove whose cause was indeed a buried hair.

Talon noir (black heel) Stigmata caused by certain operations in occupations and avocations are characteristic. The bump on the radial aspect of the middle finger of a scribe and the callused fingertips of a violinist are examples. The illustration is of punctate and ecchymotic hemorrhages in a heel of a basketball player. There is something about basketball playing in its jumps, twists, and turns that promotes this type of lesion. Its only significance is that it should not be mistaken for malignant melanoma.

Figure 742

Figure 743

Tattoos The deposition into skin of inert materials that produce colored effects may be accidental or premeditated. The usual material that enters skin accidentally is carbon from mischance like fire blast, abrasion on dirty surfaces, and stabs of sharp pencils. Figure 742 is a stripe of blue color resulting from an incised wound incurred in a fall on a tarred pavement; Figure 743 is a conventional tattoo placed by a tattoo artist. The pigments used by tattooists to produce

colors are carbon for blue and black, cinnabar or cochineal for red, cadmium salts for yellow, and cobalt salts for green. These materials are inert, but on occasion granulomas (Fig. 743) develop, especially from cinnabar. The color produced by carbon is black if placed superficially and progressively dark to light blue the deeper it is placed. The use of lasers for removal can be quite successful.

Figure 744

Clubbed nails Increased curvature of the nail plate may be due to a wide variety of causes. In this patient, the large convex nails are a hereditary anomaly and were found to be present in both father and brother. Other causes of clubbing of the nails in children include cyanotic congenital heart disease, cystic fibrosis, and chronic inflammatory bowel disease.

Figure 745

Onychodystrophy Any skin disease that affects the nail matrix may result in an abnormal nail plate. Lichen planus, sometimes without skin or mucous membrane involvement, may cause ridging and thinning of all 20 nails or pterygium formation. Psoriasis frequently results in pitting, thickening, or discoloration of the nail plate. Other etiologies include atopic dermatitis and alopecia areata. In contrast to the adult, fungal infection of the toenails and fingernails in children is a relatively rare event.

Figure 746

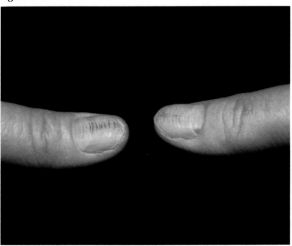

Traumatic onychodystrophy Trauma to the nail plate or nail folds can produce a wide variety of nail deformities. The one pictured here is the result of a habit tic. This common nail dystrophy is characterized by a longitudinal canal which runs down the center of the entire nail plate. It is caused by manipulation of the proximal nail fold by the index finger of the same hand.

Figure 747

Dystrophia unguis mediana canaliformis This is a rare condition of unknown etiology, which usually involves the thumb. It consists of a canal which runs near the center of the length of the nail plate. Small cracks which extend laterally from the linear canal give the appearance of an inverted fir tree. This deformity tends to resolve spontaneously over a period of months but often recurs.

Figure 748

Leukonychia totalis This is a rare nail disorder that is inherited in autosomal dominant fashion. The color of normal nail plates beyond the lunulae is largely pink from the blood in the blood vessels of the nail bed. The whiteness shown here is due to an abnormality in the nail plate. The nails may also be brittle.

Figure 749

Leukonychia striata The horizontal white streaks pictured here are the result of abnormal keratinization of the nail plate. The tendency toward leukonychia striata is sometimes inherited in autosomal dominant fashion. In other cases, it can be attributed to vigorous manicuring or to a wide variety of systemic illnesses. In many patients, there is no obvious cause, and the streaks resolve spontaneously.

Figure 750

Onycholysis (drug-induced) This word means separation (-*lysis*) of nails (*onycho*-) from nail beds. There are many causes for such a development. The commonest are mechanical. Nails worn long are frequently lifted by being snagged. Excessive soaping and soaking entailed in heavy housework promote separation. The illustration is of another cause, namely, an idiopathic response by photosensitivity in a patient who had been taking demethylchlortetracycline.

Figure 751

Discoloration of nail plates Many chemicals can discolor nail plates. Solutions of potassium permanganate and silver nitrate stain nail plates brown-purple and jet black, respectively. In the case illustrated, the stain derived from resorcinol. Such stains are harmless and can be easily removed by superficial scaling with the edge of a glass slide.

Figure 752

Figure 753

Trichotillomania This is a form of alopecia which is caused by the child's twisting or pulling of his or her own hair. This cause of hair loss is usually easy to recognize. There is often, but not always, a parental awareness of hair pulling behavior, sometimes while studying, watching television, or at bedtime. The area of hair loss is usually asymmetric and follows an irregular pattern. Examination of the involved area reveals hairs that are broken off at different lengths. There is never the total hair loss of alopecia areata or the scaling and

erythema of tinea capitis. In most cases, trichotillomania is evidence of an innocent and benign habit that is best compared to nail biting. However, trichotillomania may sometimes be evidence of more severe emotional distress. In addition, children who swallow their plucked hairs may develop a gastric trichobezoar. The daily application, by the child if possible, of petrolatum to the affected areas is a useful maneuver. It serves as a reminder to stop pulling or twirling, and it makes the hair slippery and hard to pull out.

Figure 754

Figure 755

Traumatic alopecia Another traumatic form of alopecia is due to hairstyles that feature braiding with excessive tension. The picture in Fig. 754 shows hair loss caused by a ponytail. Cornrows or excessively tight braids have a similar effect. The alopecia in this condition is limited to the line of the hair part or to the margins of the scalp. Careful examination

reveals broken hairs of varying lengths and sometimes a localized folliculitis. The application of heat or of chemicals to straighten hair will also damage the hair shafts and cause traumatic alopecia. An example of this phenomenon is illustrated in Fig. 755. For most cases of traumatic alopecia, a change in hairstyle is the only treatment that is required.

Figure 756

Figure 757

Alopecia areata The children pictured in Figs. 756 and 757 are typical of the most common presentation of alopecia areata. There is usually a history of the abrupt onset of hair loss in one or several circumscribed round or oval patches. There is no history of pruritus or scaling. The occasional association of alopecia areata with diseases like lymphocytic thyroiditis and vitiligo suggests a possible autoimmune etiology. Fortunately, spontaneous regrowth occurs in most patients over a period of 6 months to 1 year. Prognosis is less favorable in patients with more widespread disease and earlier onset. During the initial onset, parents and children should be counseled with cautious optimism, but forewarned that progression of the disorder may occur or that it may recur after a period of complete recovery. The use of topical and intralesional corticosteroids or of topical anthralin ointment seems to hasten the resolution of the process.

Figure 758

Figure 759

Alopecia areata Illustrated in Fig. 758 is ophiasis, a form of alopecia where hair loss progresses along the margin of the scalp. Figure 759 is a severe example of alopecia areata which is progressing toward alopecia totalis. Both ophiasis and extensive alopecia areata carry a poor prognosis for regrowth. The use of intralesional steroids in patients with such extensive disease is extremely painful. Topical agents which cause either an irritant or contact dermatitis of the scalp may sometimes stimulate hair growth. However, they do not seem to affect the tendency toward progression and repeated recurrences in patients with severe involvement. Certainly, alopecia areata has enormous implications for the self-image of the affected child or adolescent. Wigs are sometimes helpful. Patients and families should be advised of the availability of support groups related to this disease.

Figure 760

Alopecia universalis   This is the severest expression of the alopecia areata disease process. Complete loss of scalp hair is termed *alopecia totalis*. The patient pictured here has also lost all of his eyebrows, eyelashes, axillary, body, and pubic hair. Hence, alopecia universalis. The prognosis in this situation is particularly poor, with little chance of responding to therapy or of experiencing spontaneous recovery.

Figure 761

Alopecia areata (recovered)   This illustration is of regrowth of hair in a patch of alopecia areata. The oddity is that the regrowth was with white hair. The phenomenon is not unusual and is temporary. Eventually the regrowth will be in a color that is normal for the patient. It also frequently happens that regrown hair is temporarily of different texture. In time, assuming no relapse, completely normal color and texture supervene.

Figure 762

Histopathology of alopecia areata and trichotillomania   Alopecia areata and trichotillomania may at times be difficult to tell apart clinically. Histologically, they are readily distinguished. In alopecia areata (illustrated on the left) hair follicles become diminutive but continue to produce fine hairs. Often there is inflammation, seen here surrounding the centrally situated follicle. At high magnification one can observe mitotic activity in the matrix of the hair bulb, indicating residual

Figure 763

viability. In trichotillomania (illustrated on the right) the follicles are not reduced in size, but they no longer produce normal hair shafts. Instead one finds keratinous debris within the pilary canals, which, moreover, are no longer straight, and clumps of dark melanin pigment, seen in both the follicles. In other types of diffuse alopecia, biopsy is of little value. In conditions that terminate in permanent alopecia, scarring can be observed microscopically.

Figure 764

Figure 765

Monilethrix This word means *beaded hair* and designates a condition in which the hair varies in thickness along its length. Inheritance is autosomal dominant. The result is that the hair remains dry and brittle and fractures easily. Children with this condition may have normal neonatal hairs, but the hair that begins to grow in the second or third month of life will fracture before reaching a normal length. The condition may resolve spontaneously over time or persist into adult life.

Trichorrhexis nodosa This is another anomaly of hair growth. It is characterized by dry, fragile hair and results in patches of partial alopecia. The second word in the condition's name derives from the presence of whitish nodes along the hair shaft. These nodes are the site of breakage. This disorder is very rarely associated with argininosuccinicaciduria and mental retardation. The acquired forms are far more common and seem to be the combined result of trauma to the hair and a genetic predisposition.

Figure 766

Figure 767

Monilethrix and trichorrhexis nodosa (magnified appearance of hair shafts) Use of a hand lens or low-power magnification by microscope reveals the anomalies in the hair shafts. The upper part of the figure shows the hair in monilethrix. The nodes are strung on a thin, internodal shaft. The lower part of the picture shows the distinctive appearance of the hair in trichorrhexis nodosa. The nodes look like brushes or brooms. Breakage of hair occurs at the weak internodes of monilethrix and at the brush-like nodes of trichorrhexis nodosa.

Pili torti The title means twisted (*torti*) hairs (*pili*). The gross clinical appearance is of diffuse alopecia and dry, fragile hair. Magnification of hairs in this condition reveals spiral twists at irregular intervals along the long axes of the shafts. Pili torti is seen in association with a number of enzyme deficiencies and hereditary syndromes, including citrullinemia and Bazex syndrome. It may also be associated with sensorineural hearing loss. No effective treatment is available.

Figure 768

Figure 769

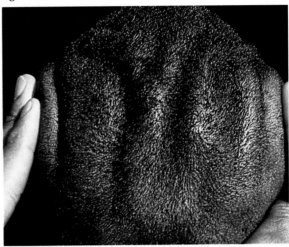

Nevoid hypertrichosis   Illustrated here is a hamartoma consisting entirely of hair follicles. A small lesion of this type is completely benign and unimportant. The presence of a patch of hypertrichosis overlying the mid-lower back, however, may be an indication of a significant underlying neurologic abnormality. The so-called faun tail nevus may signal the presence of spina bifida occulta, diastemetomyelia, or duplication or tethering of the spinal cord. A thorough neurologic investigation is warranted in such cases.

Cutis verticis gyrata   Scalp skin sometimes develops redundantly as a congenital anomaly or in association with a disease like acromegaly. The consequence is furrowed wrinkling of hyperplastic skin in a pattern that suggests the puzzled pate of a bulldog, in whom the condition is natural. There are cases that are so extreme that hygiene of the scalp is difficult and the cosmetic appearance justifiably disturbing. Plastic surgery is a reasonable treatment.

26

Miscellaneous Anomalies

Figure 770

Figure 771

Aplasia cutis congenita Among the many hazards of intra-uterine development and sojourn is failure at times to achieve complete congenital integrity of the integument. It sometimes happens that a child is born with a superficial erosion, as in Fig. 770, or an ulcer, as in Fig. 771. The vertex of the scalp is a common place for the phenomenon to occur; the hands, face, and points over bony prominences are also susceptible. Aplasia cutis congenita is frequently a benign event of only cosmetic importance and in most cases the etiology is not established. However, epidermolysis bullosa, placental in-farction, teratogens, and some chromosome deletions and trisomies are occasionally implicated as causes. A lesion may be directly adjacent to an epidermal nevus or nevus sebaceus, or it may overlie a defect in the bone. More significant underlying anomalies are meningomyeloceles, spinal dys-raphisms, and various cerebral malformations. Hemorrhage and secondary infection may occur, requiring emergency treatment. The combination of aplasia cutis congenita and distal limb reduction is an additional inherited disorder.

Figure 772

Figure 773

Aplasia cutis congenita These are examples of cutaneous aplasias that have healed into parchment-like scars. This process may occur in utero or shortly after birth. Figure 772 pictures a lesion that healed postpartum. Note that the defect involved the full thickness of skin and resulted in destruction of the pilar adnexa. In consequence, the scar, healed by secondary intention, is quite bald. In Fig. 773 the same sort of thing is shown on the dorsum of the hand and parts adjacent; it could pass as a scar consequent to an ordinary thermal burn. Aside from the cosmetic defect, the scars of healed congenital aplasias are good and ordinarily serve normal function well enough. In a place like the scalp, alopecic scars of large size that cannot be adequately covered by surrounding hair can be restored to near normal by hair transplants, which fortunately take quite well. In other places, plastic revision could correct undesirable sequelae such as adhesions, if such have occurred.

Figure 774

Figure 775

Supernumerary digits   Supernumerary digits, like other supernumerary structures, come in all degrees of development, from merest suggestion to nearly full reduplication. The figure shows a fairly well-developed extra digit containing bones, musculature, and nerves and situated in a common site just beyond the last natural finger. More commonly, the vestige consists of a small nubbin of soft tissue in the same location. Treatment is by surgical excision.

Amputation neuroma   Although surgical removal of a supernumerary digit is a technically simple operation, a rare complication is illustrated here. It is an amputation neuroma, a knot of neural tissue formed in the wound of an operation for removal of a structure that had nerves within it. Such a lesion can be tender to touch, spontaneously painful, and possibly productive of phantom symptoms. Reexcision is obviously necessary.

Figure 776

Figure 777

Histopathology of amputation neuroma   Small papules found at birth on the ulnar aspect of the fifth finger are remnants of supernumerary digits (pedunculated postminimi). Similar papules may develop after attempted surgical ablation of supernumerary digits. They show the same histopathology as digital traumatic neuromas regardless of cause. In the photomicrograph, one sees marked proliferation of nerves in dense collagenous stroma and Wagner-Meissner corpuscles in the dermal papillae.

Supernumerary nipple   Supernumerary nipples are exceedingly common in both sexes. In women, more than mere nipples, considerable mammary glands may develop along the "milk lines" from axillae to pubes. In males, one supernumerary nipple and a set of two are common enough; two, even three, complete pairs are still not rare. The degree of development may be from vestiges that could be taken for common pigmented moles to well-developed ones like those pictured.

Figure 778

Figure 779

Auricular tags Supernumerary vestiges of the external structures of ears are common. Accessory tragi and auricular tags with or without communication to deeper structures may be deceptively simple. The ones in Fig. 778 are probably harmless nubs of tissue that could be sliced off and their bases delicately electrodesiccated. Should that be all there is, the cosmetic result would be fine. Sometimes, however, such structures bear cartilage within them and have communication to un-

certain depths toward the more important structures in the external canal or middle ear. In Fig. 779 there is a bit of reduplicated auricular tissue that had been displaced onto the neck. Again, the anomalous tissue could be easily excised if it had no communication deeper and upward. In the latter event, more thorough dissection of the entire structure would be required. It is not an office procedure.

Figure 780

Figure 781

Histopathology of accessory tragi Papules near the normal tragus of the ear are usually rudimentary, accessory tragi. In such lesions, one sees epidermis, from which are derived many fine hair-producing follicles. Deep to the dermis, a layer of adipose tissue surrounding a central core of cartilage may often be found. Even if a cartilaginous core is not present, the other features mentioned are sufficient to distinguish an accessory tragus from a soft fibroma.

Dental sinus Infection at or around the apex of a tooth may become an abscess that burrows toward exit on the skin. The simplest situation is a channel from a tooth in the lower jaw onto the skin over the mandible, on the underside of the chin or jaw or on the neck. The presenting lesion may appear, like the one pictured, at the junction of jaw and neck, as a superficial pyoderma or an infected cyst. Simple drainage and topical antisepsis fail to cure. Discovery and extirpation of the internal source are required.

Figure 782

Figure 783

Branchial-cleft cysts The embryogenesis of the head and neck must be a fetus's nightmare. Because so many structures have to come together perfectly from both sides, it is remarkable that they ever do. But they almost always do. Failure of perfect coaptation is to be expected on occasion. Cleft palate and cleft lips are well known and easily recognizable. More subtle is failure of perfect development of the branchial arches. The usual clinical lesion is an insignificant-looking papule or small cystic mass on one side of the neck, anteriorly off center. In Fig. 782 there is such a lesion. Figure 783 shows a much rarer bilateral anomaly of this nature. Surgical ablation of such embryonic errors is not easy. It takes an operator skilled in head and neck surgery to trace out the unexpected twists and turns of such cysts and sinuses from important structures of the region.

Figure 784

Figure 785

Thyroglossal cyst This is another example of a dysraphism of midline structures. Thyroglossal cysts and fistulas are similar in appearance to branchial cleft malformations but are usually midline and located near the hyoid bone. These lesions may become complicated by enlargement or secondary infection. Careful excision is recommended.

Sucking blister The oval blister pictured here was present at birth and is a result of normal sucking behavior in utero. Sucking blisters are fairly common and are usually located on the forearm, wrist, or hand. They most often are solitary and involve only one upper extremity. However, lesions involving both hands, or even involving a foot, are sometimes seen. The sucking blister resolves spontaneously as soon as bottle or breast is offered as a dietary substitute.

Figure 786

Figure 787

Anomalies of umbilical maldevelopment A number of developmental abnormalities may accompany an umbilicus with abnormal appearance. Figure 786 shows an umbilicus that gives exit to a patent urachus. The persistent urachus is due to failure of closure of the allantoic duct. This diagnosis is usually suggested by the presence of a clear liquid discharge

from the umbilicus. The bright red polyp in Fig. 787 is a remnant of the distal portion of the omphalomesenteric duct. The mucosal lining of this lesion may represent small intestine, stomach, or colon. Fistulas of the duct, Meckel's diverticulum, and ileal prolapse may accompany this malformation. Treatment in all cases is surgical.

Figure 788

Figure 789

Histopathology of omphalomesenteric duct remnant Of all possible umbilical anomalies, the one related to the gastrointestinal tract is usually missed clinically but is easily diagnosed microscopically. Therefore, persistent abnormalities on and around the umbilicus should be biopsied. Here one sees a sessile lesion covered by stratified squamous epithelium and bearing two foci of enteral epithelium near the summit. There are prominent glands and cystic structures within the lesion.

Umbilical granuloma It is normal for the umbilical cord to separate about 6 to 8 days after birth and for the resulting wound to heal within 2 weeks. This process may be slowed by a mild infection at the base of the cord, and is sometimes complicated by the invasion of true pathogenic organisms. Pictured here is the formation of heaped-up granulation tissue at and in the umbilicus—the so-called umbilical granuloma. Treatment by repeated cauterization with silver nitrate is usually successful.

Figure 790

The appearance of the lips of suckling infants The cheeks and lips of neonates are normally well adapted for suckling. The cheeks have fat-padded musculature to produce strong suction, and the lips have surface markings that help to hold a nipple firmly. In the picture one sees a tubercle in the center of the upper lip and serrations to each side of it and on the entire surface of the lower lip. In feeding, these formations deepen and make grip all the firmer.

Figure 791

Fordyce's condition The face abounds in sebaceous glands. Normally their distribution stops sharply at the junction of the skin and vermilion of the lips. Commonly, however, ectopic sebaceous glands are found within the lips under the vermilion and sometimes within the oral mucosa of the lips and even in the buccal mucosa. The condition is harmless and may have been present long before the patient or parents have become aware of it. No treatment is required or available.

Figure 792

Geographic tongue There is a peculiar condition of the tongue which takes the form of denudations of the lingual surface in patches of redness that shift in position from time to time over hours and days. The cause of the condition is not known; there may be some relationship to psoriasis. No treatment is effective. The condition is largely asymptomatic except for slight tingling when sharp food is taken.

Figure 793

Mucocele The lower lip is studded with cells that produce mucus. Mucoceles are cysts deriving from such cells. They appear as papules that are visibly and palpably filled with highly viscous fluid. They are harmless and asymptomatic but require extirpation because they make themselves felt when within the mouth and are cosmetically objectionable when on the lips. When reasonably small, like the one pictured, electrodesiccation and curettage are sufficient; larger lesions may require scalpel surgery.

Index

Index

This index has been compiled from the text of the legends, and the reference numbers are the figure numbers.